AF887564

ONKOLOGIE

Supplement 1 zu Band 15, April 1992

Internationale Zeitschrift für Krebsforschung und -behandlung

Impressum

Offizielles Organ der Deutschen Gesellschaft für Hämatologie und Onkologie, der Österreichischen Gesellschaft für Hämatologie und Onkologie, der Österreichischen Krebsgesellschaft – Krebsliga unter Fortführung der «Österreichischen Zeitung für Onkologie»

Schriftleitung

H. Huber, Innsbruck
W. Queißer, Mannheim

Fachschriftleitung

W. E. Berdel, Berlin
E. Dühmke, Göttingen
N. Jaeger, Hildesheim
M. Kaufmann, Heidelberg
P. Schlag, Heidelberg

Wissenschaftlicher Beirat

W. E. Berdel, Berlin
V. Diehl, Köln
C. Dittrich, Wien
P. Drings, Heidelberg
E. Dühmke, Göttingen
H. H. Fiebig, Freiburg
A. Gläser, Halle
R. Hartenstein, München
K. Havemann, Marburg
K. P. Hellriegel, Berlin
R. Herrmann, Basel
H .W. von Heyden, Einbeck
D. Hoelzer, Frankfurt / M.
J. H. Holzner, Wien
H. Huber, Innsbruck
H. J. Illiger, Oldenburg
N. Jaeger, Hildesheim
R. Jakesz, Wien
M. Kaufmann, Heidelberg
U. R. Kleeberg, Hamburg
B. Kornhuber, Frankfurt / M.
H. Löffler, Kiel
H. Ludwig, Wien
U. Mohr, Hannover
K. Munk, Heidelberg
G. A. Nagel, Vitikon-Zürich
A. Pfleiderer, Freiburg
F. Porzsolt, Ulm
K. Possinger, München
W. Queißer, Mannheim
P. Schlag, Heidelberg
H.-J. Schmoll, Hannover
M. Schröder, Kassel
S. Seeber, Essen
W. Vahlensieck, Bonn
H. W. Waclawiczek, Salzburg
M. Wannenmacher, Heidelberg
H. J. Weh, Hamburg
W. Wilmanns, München

Anzeigen
S. Karger Verlag für Medizin und Naturwissenschaften GmbH,
Postfach 1724, W-8034 Germering, Telefon (0 89) 84 30 35.
Gültig ist die Preisliste Nr. 6 vom 1. 10. 1990.

Für den Inhalt außerhalb des redaktionellen Teiles (insbesondere Anzeigen, Industrieinformationen, Pressezitate und Kongreßinformationen usw.) übernehmen Schriftleitung, Beirat und Verlag keine Gewähr.

Eine Markenbezeichnung kann warenzeichengeschützt sein, auch wenn bei Ihrer Verwendung in dieser Zeitschrift das Zeichen ® oder ein anderer Hinweis auf etwa bestehende Schutzrechte fehlen sollte. Für Satzfehler, insbesondere bei Dosierungsangaben, wird keine Gewähr übernommen.

Alle Rechte, insbesondere das Recht der Vervielfältigung und Mikrokopie sowie der Übersetzung vorbehalten. Nachdruck, auch auszugsweise, nur mit Genehmigung des Verlages. Fotokopien dürfen nur für den persönlichen Gebrauch als Einzelkopien hergestellt werden. Jede im Bereich eines gewerblichen Unternehmens zulässig hergestellte oder benutzte Kopie dient gewerblichen Zwecken gem. § 54(2) UrhG und verpflichtet zur Gebührenzahlung an die Verwertungsgesellschaft WORT, Abt. VG Wissenschaft, Goethestr. 49, W-8000 München 2.

© Copyright 1992 by S. Karger
Verlag für Medizin und Naturwissenschaften GmbH,
Postfach 1724,
W-8034 Germering (BRD)

ISBN 3-8055-5637-3

Verlagsleitung: Manfred R. Just
Redaktionsassistenz: Anne Schieber
Anzeigenverkauf: Marlene Scholz
Anzeigenverwaltung: Eva M. Lindenau
Herstellung: Horst H. Bruch
Vertrieb: Gabriela Taube

Satz und Druck: Bonitas-Bauer, Grafischer Betrieb,
Max-von-Laue-Str. 31, W-8700 Würzburg.

Ladenpreis dieses Sonderheftes DM 28,- inkl. MwSt.:
Abonnenten erhalten es unberechnet.

Bezugspreis der Zeitschrift:
Für Jahrgang 14, 1991, DM 148,– / öS 1036,– / SFr 116,–.
1 Einzelheft kostet DM 28,– / öS 196,– / SFr 22,– einschließlich MwSt., zuzüglich Postgebühren.

KARGER

Supplement 1 zu Band 15, April 1992

ONKOLOGIE

Internationale Zeitschrift für Krebsforschung und -behandlung

Contents

2nd Frankfurt International Cytokine Symposium
June 25–27, 1992, Frankfurt am Main,
Federal Republic of Germany

Chairpersons:
L. Bergmann
P. S. Mitrou
Department of Hematology/Oncology
J.W. Goethe-University
W-6000 Frankfurt am Main 1
Federal Republic of Germany

Scientific Committee:
L. Bergmann, Frankfurt/Main
C. Huber, Mainz
P. S. Mitrou, Frankfurt/Main
N. Niederle, Leverkusen

Location:
Steigenberger Hotel «Frankfurter Hof»
Kaiserplatz
W-6000 Frankfurt/Main 1
Federal Republic of Germany

Bibliographischer Hinweis: Inhaltsverzeichnisse dieser Zeitschrift erscheinen regelmäßig in *current contents*® sowie in anderen bibliographischen Diensten.

Date	Time	Scientific Program
Wednesday June 24, 1992	19.30 - 21.30	Welcome buffet dinner (Frankfurter Hof)
Thursday June 24, 1992	8.30 - 10.20	Cytokine network and receptors (Invited lectures, L-1 - L-3)
	10.20 - 10.50	Coffee break
	10.50 - 13.00	Interferons in CML and lymphomas (Invited lectures, L-4 - L-8)
	13.00 - 14.30	Lunch
	14.30 - 16.30	Interferons and TNF in malignancies (Invited lectures, L-9 - L-12)
	16.30 - 16.50	Coffee break
	16.50 - 18.30	Free communications (T-1 - T-10)
	18.30 - 19.00	Main lecture (L-13)
Friday June 26, 1992	8.30 - 10.30	IL-2 and cytotoxic mechanisms (Invited lectures, L-14 - L-17)
	10.30 - 10.45	Coffee break
	10.45 - 12.15	Combinations of cytokines and gene transfer (Invited lectures, L-18 - L-20)
	12.15 - 13.15	Lunch
	13.15 - 14.30	Poster discussion (P-1 - P-44)
	14.30 - 16.20	Free communication (F-1 - F-11)
	16.20 - 16.45	Coffee break
	16.45 - 18.15	Free communication (F-12 - F-20)
	18.30 - 19.00	Main lecture (L-21)
	20.00	Dinner party (Frankfurter Hof)
Saturday June 27, 1992	8.30 - 10.30	IL-2 in leukemia (Invited lectures, L-22 - L-26)
	10.30 - 11.00	Coffee break
	11.00 - 14.30	Biological functions of various cytokines and adhesion molecules (Invited lectures, L-27 - L-33)

Onkologie 1992;15(suppl 1):1-35

2nd Frankfurt International Cytokine Symposium
organized by the
Cancer Center Frankfurt am Main
and the
German Cancer Society
and the
Society for Medical Oncology

Frankfurt am Main, Federal Republic of Germany, June 25 - 27, 1992

Abstracts

Invited Lectures

L1 - L3 missing

L-4

Combinations of IFN-Alpha with other Cytokines as Initial and Second-line Therapy of Chronic Myeloid Leukemia (CML)

O. Kloke
Dept. of Internal Medicine (Cancer Research), Essen

IFN-alpha has shown the capacity to suppress the neoplastic Ph-positive cell clone of CML. A significant cytogenetic improvement, however, is confined to a minority of patients treated. Therefore, the search for a combination treatment that enhances the activity of IFN-alpha is warranted.
We have studied combinations of IFN-alpha with other cytokines both in first-line treatment of CML and in patients with IFN-alpha-resistant disease. Combined administration of IFN's alpha and gamma was found to induce a hematologic remission in individual patients resistant to either of the IFN's alone. Furthermore, the addition of TNF which by itself had no cytoreductive activity led to a hematologic improvement in 5/6 patients with IFN-alpha-resistant CML. Data thus indicate a role for IFN-gamma and TNF in the modification of IFN-alpha resistance. Involving patients with previously untreated CML, the combination of IFN-alpha and low-dose IFN-gamma was compared, in a randomized study, with single-agent IFN-alpha. Analysis of 51 patients enrolled failed to reveal an enhancement of IFN-alpha effectiveness in fist-line therapy. In summary, it remains unclear at present whether the addition of other cytokines offers in chance to enhance the antileukemic action of IFN-alpha in CML.

L-5 missing

L-6

Interferon alpha (IFN) in the Treatment of Chronic Myelogenous Leukemia (CML): Results of a Randomized Multicenter Trial in Germany

R. Hehlmann, H. Heimpel, H.-J. Kolb, H. Ansari, B. Heinze, T. Buhr, D. K. Hossfeld, M. Grießhammer, P. D. Wickramanayake, U. Essers, C. Falge, L. Bergmann, W. Queißer, H. Pralle, H. Löffler, P. Meyer, A. Hochhaus, P. v. Wussow, A. Georgii, J. Hasford and the German CML-Study-Group
III. Med. Klinik Mannheim, Universität Heidelberg, Mannheim

Recent developments of INF-therapy in CML are illustrated by the results of a controlled multicenter trial in Germany. From

July 1983 to January 1991 a total of 624 CML-patients were randomized to compare the effects of hydroxyurea, interferon alpha (IFN), and busulfan on duration of chronic phase, surival and outcome of bone marrow transplantation (BMT). Further goals include the determination of prognostic parameters. 89% of the patients were Ph-positive (+). 11% had additonal chromosome aberrations. The median survival of Ph+ patients by now is 4.1 years, that of Ph- patients 1.2 years. Ph-negative patients tend to have lower white blood cell (103.000 vs. 168.000) and platelet counts (3700.000 vs. 495.000). Prospectively evaluated age, organomegaly related symptoms, Karnofsky index, extramedullary manifestations, erythroblasts and percent of circulating blasts proved to be of prognostic significance. A prognostic score (score 1) was determined which was superior to Sokal's score in the study population. 164 patients were randomized to receive IFN. In 50 patients (30%) IFN had to be terminated because of adverse effects, therapy resistance or other reasons. Most frequent adverse events were flu-like symptoms in 74%, gastrointestinal symptoms in 52%, and neurologic-psychiatric symptoms in 30% of patients. Reduction of the Ph-chromosome was observed in 14% of evaluable patients. In 3 patients complete cytogenetic remissions were observed. Clinically relevant neutralizing antibodies were detected in 9 cases. 233 patients were randomized to receive hydroxyurea. In this group the lowest number of adverse effects is being observed. BMT was done in 53 study patients (15 pretreated with busulfan, 21 with hydroxyurea, 17 with IFN). 5-year survival after BMT is 60%. No survival advantage can be recognized for any pretreatment group. No difference of survival is detectable for BMT carried out during the first three years of the chronic phase, whereas survival after BMT in accelerated phase and in patients with marrow fibrosis is clearly inferior. The study results will allow statements as to the advantages or disadvantages of the use of busulfan, hydroxyurea and IFN in the treatment of CML as well as to the reliability of prognostic markers.

L-7

Clinical Significance of Interferons in the Treatment of Malignant Lymphomas

M. Freund
Dept. of Hematology and Oncology, Hannover Medical School

Interferon alpha (IFN α) is a therapeutic principe with well established activity in malignant Non-Hodgkin's lymphomas. The most favorable results have been achieved in low grade malignant histologies. Objective responses of about 40% have been reported in patients with nodular histology (mostly centrocytic-centroblastic according to the Kiel classification). There are some indications for a dose-response relationship but evidence from randomized studies is still missing. In advanced chronic lymphocytic leukemia, responses have been noted in 15% of patients only. There are data indicating a possible *in vitro* growth-stimulation of CLL-cells by IFN α with a response rate of 70 percent. Complete response have not been reported with IFN α in CLL but can be achieved by new powerful cytotoxic drugs. Additionally the prognosis of CLL in the early stages is favorable. The impact of IFN α in early CLL is still open. There are controversial data on the treatment of cutaneous T-cell lymphoma and mycosis fungoides with IFN α. Based on pooled published data, the overall response-rate is about 40%. High-grade malignant Non-Hodgkin's lymphomas have been treated with high doses of IFN α with an overall remission-rate of 15 percent. In most cases, remissions have been short.
The effectivity of IFN α as a monotherapy is comparable to that of some cytotoxic agents. Despite this fact is final place in the therapeutic strategy is controversial. The combination of IFN α with alkylating agents is very effectively inducing remissions in low grade NHL, but additional hematoxicity may evolve. In other studies IFN α is given for maintenance after conventional chemotherapy-induction. There is some evidence that the remission duration may be improved. However, an improvement of survival still has to be demonstrated.

L-8

Interferon-alpha in the Treatment of B-Cell Chronic Lymphocytic Leukemia

E. Thiel
Dept. of Hematology and Oncology, Klinikum Steglitz, Free University, Berlin

In pilot studies, interferon-alpha (IFN-α) was found to be effective in chronic lymphocytic leukemia of B-cell type (B-CLL). Efficacy of IFN-a was reported to be higher in early stage B-CLL than in advanced stages. It has been shown to reduce the number of circulating leukemic cells, the size of enlarged lymphnodes and of liver and spleen, respectively. Moreover, serum immunoglobulin levels may increase during treatment with IFN-α. Various attempts have been made to elucidate mechanisms of action of IFN-α in B-CLL. One possible mode of action may be the interruption of the TNF-α associated autocrine growth by mRNA damage, which is caused by IFN-α inducible ribonucleases. These considerations and experiences from pilot studies prompted us to initiate a risk factor adapted randomized multicenter study on IFN-α in early stage B-CLL. Only previously untreated patients with Binet stage A disease and at high risk for progression (diffuse bone marrow infiltration, plus short lymphocyte doubling time and/or high levels of serum thymidinkinase) are randomized for treatment with IFN-α or observation. Patients without risk factors serve as controls. Up to now, 110 patients were included into the study. Preliminary results seem to confirm the relevance of the risk factors and provide evidence, that IFN-α may maintain freedom from progression and chemotherapy. An updated survey of the trial will be presented.

L-9

Treatment Results in Hairy Cell Leukemia with Interferon alpha

H. Pralle
Gießen

Since 1984, the observation of five remission in six patients with hairy cell leukemia (HCL) treated by natural Interferon (IFN_{leu}) in a low-dose schedule, has given rise to a series of multicenter trials. The coincident availability of 3 subtypes of hr Ifn-alpha 2 initiated three major trials. The results they came up with were in principle identical. The patients improved gradually over a period of several weeks with regression of splenomegaly, improvement of thrombocytes and hemoglobin and a steadily increasing number of granulocytes and even monocytes after several months. Clearance of bone marrow was observed in several pa-

tients, beginning after the fourth month at the earliest, and then gradually increasing until the years three and four. The application schedule proved very safe. It was only during the first three or four months that the patients remained prone to various bacterial, microbacterial and fungal infections. According to the American study, after this period, their improved general performance status and response to infectious challenges resulted in an overall survival rate of 91% after the fourth year.
Patients relapsed when the drug was withdrawn after 8-22 months. It proved possible to reintroduce remissions by again administering the same subtype and dose of hrIFN.
A minor percentage of patients developed neutralizing antibodies against hrIfN and lost its efficacy. Two observations were made in the treatment following. The antibodies could be circumvented most easily by IfN_{leu}. On the other hand, the neutralizing capacity of the antibodies diminished after several weeks of continuous treatment with the same type of Ifn declining to very low levels.
The introduction of Ifn alpha in HCL led to several important observations concerning the immunomodulation of the host and on molecular events in HC. Unfortunately, until now none of the discoveries offered an explanation for the astounding clinical efficacy.

L-10

Modulation of the Activity of Cytotoxic Drugs by Interferons in the Treatment of Cancer

S. Wadler, E. L. Schwartz
Albert Einstein Cancer Center and Montefiore Medical Center, New York, USA

The interferons (IFNs) are a family of multifunctional cytokines with cytotoxic and negative growth regulatory effects on human cancer cells. IFNs have been shown to modulate the activity of over 20 different cytotoxic drugs in vitro; however, incorporation of these IFN/drug combinations into the clinical armamentarium has proven difficult. The combination of IFN and 5-fluorouracil (5FU) has been successfully exploited in various phase I and phase II studies and has entered phase III trials in the United States and Europa for the treatment of colorectal carcinoma. Clinical and preclinical studies have been initiated to attempt to elucidate the mechanism of interaction of these two agents, and the findings from these studies illustrade the complexity of the interaction between biologic and cytotoxic agents. For example, 4/5 pharmacokinetic studies have demonstrated that IFN can augment serum levels of 5FU by up to 64-fold. In one of these studies, enhancement of pharmacokinetic effects occured at doses of IFN as low as 100,000 U. At the cellular level, IFN augments anabolism of 5FU to its active metabolite, fluorodeoxyuridylate (FdUMP), by augmenting the activity of the anabolic enzyme, thymidine phosphorylase. Furthermore, IFN inhibits transcription of the 5FU target enzyme, thymidylate synthase (TS), resultind in a reversal of the 5FU-stimulated increase in TS levels observed following exposure of cells to the fluoropyrimidine. This results in a decrease in TS activity in the treated cell lines. The critical locus for the synergy between 5FU and IFN remains to be defined, and the interaction may be multifactorial or alternatively may differ among various systems. Combinations of IFNs and cytotoxic drugs other than 5FU also appear promising. For example, the combination of IFN/DTIC is active in melanoma and prolonged survival in one randomized study, and the combination of IFN/cisplatin is active in squamous cell carcinomas of the lung, and head and neck.

L-11

Isolated Limp Perfusion with High Dose Tumor Necrosis Factor-α, Gamma-Interferon and Melphalan for Irresectable Melanomas or Soft Tissue Sarcomas

A. M. M. Eggermont[a], D. Liénard[c], H. Schraffordt Koops[b], F. J. Lejeune[c]
[a] Rotterdam Cancer Institut, Netherlands
[b] University Hospital Groningen, Netherlands
[c] CPO-CHUV, Lausanne, Switzerland

Recently Lejeune's group reported a very high CR rate of > 80% in 19 melanoma stage III a/ab and 4 soft tissue sarcoma patients (pts) after isolated limb perfusion (ILP) with high dose TNF + IFN + Melphalan (J Clin Oncol 10:52-60, 1992). In our institutions, 70 patients have now been treated.
Material and Methods: 50 Patients with stage III melanoma and 20 pts with irresectable soft tissue sarcomas of the leg (17) or arm (3) have been treated. Patients received .2 mg IFN s.c. on the 2 days prior to the ILP. ILP consisted of a 1 ½ hour long perfusion with .2 mg IFN, 4 mg TNF (leg) or 2 mg TNF (arm), and 10-13 mg/l limb volume of Melphalan at 39-40 °C.
Results: 46/50 melanoma patients had a CR (92%), 4 a PR (8%). Median duration of response 14+ months. In 17/20 (85%) sarcoma patient limb salvage has been achieved. In 8 patients a CR was obtained and in 7 patients a PR making the tumor resectable; in 2 patients a PR was seen in the presence of lung metastases. Toxicity has been severe (shock, ARDS, renal failure) in some patients with leakage > 10%, with 2 treatment related deaths. In most patients (leakage 1-2%) only fever with chills and mild hypotension occurred. Local toxicity was the same as after ILP with Melphalan alone.
Conclusion: Isolated limb perfusion with high dose TNF, IFN and Melphalan is very effective in achieving limb salvage in patients with melanoma stage III or irresectable soft tissue sarcoma.

L-12 - L-13 missing

L-14

Endocrinologic Principles in the Therapeutic Use of Interleukin-2

Kendall A. Smith
Dartmouth Medical School, Hanover, NH, USA

Interleukin 2 (IL-2), a cytokine produced by antigen-activated T cells promotes the proliferation and differentiation of all lymphoid cells, and is critical for the generation of both cell-mediated immunity and humoral immunity. It is also necessary for both a primary and secondary immune response and the generation of immunologic memory. Therefore, IL-2 should be useful as an immune stimulant, particularly for patients with infectious diseases, AIDS, and perhaps selected cancers.
The key to the rational use of IL-2 as an immune stimulant is the IL-2 receptor (IL-2R). The IL-2R consists of 2 chains, of 55.000 Da (p55) and 75.000 (p75). When both chains are expressed

simultaneously, high affinity (Kd=10^{-11}M) heterodimeric receptors are formed. Expressed singly, both chains bind IL-2 with much lower affinity (p75 Kd=10^{-9}M; p55 Kd=10^{-8}M). T cells and B cells only express functional, high affinity IL-2Rs transiently, and only after antigen stimulation. By comparison, NK cells express p75 chains constitutively. Since the Kd for binding to isolated p75 is 100-fold lower than for IL-2 binding to the high affinity IL-2Rs, 100-fold higher concentrations of IL-2 are necessary to trigger NK cells, compared to activated T cells or B cells.

NK cells make up ~ 10% of all circulating mononuclear cells. Given a normal WBC count, ~ 10^9 NK cells are circulating, all responsive to high concentrations of IL-2. When triggered by IL-2, NK cells secrete a characteristic cytokine profile, which includes IFN-γ, GM-CSF and TNF-α. These cytokines are all potent monocyte stimulants, and IL-1, IL-6, IL-8 and TNF-α are known to be released by activated monocytes. If IL-2 is given in high doses (> 1 mg/day), plasma concentrations of IL-2 exceed 1nM, resulting in saturation of a significant number of receptors on NK cells. Therefore, systemic toxicity, is attributable to the cytokines released by NK cells and monocytes. In lower doses (20-50 μg/day), IL-2 given parenterally (IV, SQ, ID) results in lower plasma concentrations ($\leq$ 100 pM), sufficient to saturate high affinity IL-2Rs on antigen-activated T cells and B cells and ~ 10% of NK cells.

Rational immunotherapy with immunostimulatory cytokines depends upon establishing the therapeutic index, and knowledge of the distribution and binding characteristics of the cytokine receptors. It is important to know whether a given cytokine stimulates the release of additional cytokines, and whether these cytokines are responsible for toxic or therapeutic effects.

L-15

Triggers and Activation Signals Involved in Oncolytic Function of NK and T Cells

Eva Lotzová

University of Texas, M.D. Anderson Cancer Center, Houston, TX, USA

An increasing evidence indicates that the immunotherapeutic approaches with interleukin-2 (IL-2) activated lymphocytes are not optimal. Additionally, *in vitro* data demonstrates that many fresh tumor cells display low susceptibility or are resistant to IL-2 activated lymphocytes. Therefore, we investigated the signals involved in activation of highly oncolytic cells against fresh acute myelogenous leukemia (AML) blasts. These studies demonstrated that simultaneous activation of peripheral blood or bone marrow lymphocytes with IL-2 and irradiated AML blasts or tumor cell lines, resulted in induction of cytotoxic activity against highly resistant AML targets. This approach also resulted in increased proliferative activity of cytotoxic cells, indicating a possibility to grow these cells more effectively *in vitro*. Characterization studies showed that NK cells as well as T cells were responsive to tumorinducted stimulataory signal, indicating the possibility to trigger selectively the oncolytic activity of NK cells or T cells against the tumors with preference for either of these populations. Both the induction of cytotoxicity and proliferation was dependent on cell-to-cell contact, and was not induced by soluble factors. It is of interest to note that allogeneic as well as autologous AML blasts were effective in signalling the oncolytic effect; this opsens a possiblity to use the allogeneic AML blasts for stimulation of oncolytic lymphocytes when autologous blasts are not available or are suppressive for autologous cytotoxic lymphocytes. The therapeutic possibilitites of these observations will be discussed.

L-16

Lysis Mediated by Cytolytic T Lymphocytes

Jürg Tschopp

Institute of Biochemistry, University of Lausanne, Epalinges, Switzerland

Upon activation, circulating T lymphocytes may differentiate into cytolytic T cells (CTL), containing characteristic granules. Triggering of the TCR/CD3 complex results in granule redistribution and there is clear evidence that delivery of lytic components by degranulation is an effective mechanism for target cell destruction.

Perforin, granzymes and proteoglycans are the major components present in granules. Perforin is thought to bind to the target cell membrane and assemble into multimeric lesions.

Murine CTL contain seven highly homologous serine esterases termed granzymes A-G; human CTL harbor 3 granzymes. Their role in the lethal hit delivery is unknown, although granzyme A and B may be involved in the DNA breakdown of the target cells. Targets are lysed by an apoptotic mechanism, apparently by inducing the disintegration of target cell nuclear DNA in nucleosome-sized fragments, for which a Ca^{2+} -Mg^{2+} dependent endonuclease has been postulated.

When this nuclease activity is extracted from isolated nuclei of target cells, it induces a latter pattern of DNA fragments characteristic for apoptosis. We were able to immunoprecipitate the nuclease activity with antibodies to DNAse I. Nuclei of COS cells in which DNAse I was transiently expressed displayed the ladder forming activity. Immunohistochemical localisation showed its presence in the endoplasmic reticulum. The pathway of access to the nucleus of DNAse I during CTL-mediated cytolysis remains to be defined.

L-17 missing

L-18

Combination of IL–2 with other Cytokines in Cancer Treatment. Rationale and Clinical Results

L. Bergmann

Div. of Hematology, J. W. Goethe University, Frankfurt/Main

Interleukin-2 (Il-2) alone has been shown to have some efficacy in a few human malignancies, prodominantly in renal cell cancer (RCC) and malignant melanoma (MM). Attemps to increase the antitumoral activity of lymphokine activated killer (LAK) cells by additional transfer of in vitro activated autologous cytotoxic cells (adoptive immunotherapy, AI) improved the response rate especially in RCC. In MM, so-called tumor-infiltrating lymphocytes (TILs) were propagated and transferred to patients with remarkable results. However, totally to clinical results remain unsatisfactory and the adoptive immunotherapy or TILs are expensive and time consuming.

To improve Il-2 therapy, combinations with other cytokines may be an interesting alternative. The results of in vitro investigations and animal models combining Il-2 with other cytokines are heterogeneous and depend from the study design. Here, it has to be taken into consideration that Il-2 itself induces a cytokine cascade with the induction of high amounts of endogeneous TNF-α, IFN-γ and Il-6 in vitro and in vivo. Additionally, an increase of m RNA for Il-2 in MNC was noted after exogeneous administration of Il-2. These data suggest that the addition of these secondary induced cytokines into therapy schedules may lack any positive effect. IFN-α, however, ist not induced by Il-2 and was shown to act synergistically on activation of cytotoxic cells in vitro. In vivo, the combination of IFN-α and Il-2 improved the clinical results in RCC, wereby the effect in MM ist not yet confirmed. In vitro recent reports indicate a benefit of the combination of Il-4 with Il-2 in the propagation of TILs. An interesting point is the modulation of possible negative regulating cytokines on LAK-induction or tumor cell growth as TGF-β. Our data suggest Il-2 to be an inhibitor of TGF-β.

L-19

Development of Live Tumor Vaccines using Retroviral Vectors for Transfer of Suicide Genes and Cytokines

Craig A. Mullen, R. Michael Blaese
Metabolism Branch, DCBDC, National Cancer Institute, NIH, Bethesda, MD, USA

Our goal is the development of live attenuated tumor vaccines for the adjuvant immunotherapy of cancer. Retroviral vectors containing the cytosine deaminase (CD) gene (Mullen et al: PNAS 89:33) or the murine IL-6 gene were constructed. CD functions as a suicide gene as it confers selective lethal sensitivity to the relatively nontoxic drug 5-fluorocytosine (5FC). Murine fibrosarcoma or adenocarcinoma cells were transduced with these vectors, cloned and gene expression assayed. *In vitro* cells expressing CD converted 5FC to 5-fluoroucil (5FU) and were killed, while IL-6 transduced cells secreted a 20 U IL-6/10^5 cells/24 h. Normal syngeneic mice were injected with the engineered tumors and those receiving CD+ tumors also received a 2 wk course of intraperitoneal 5FC (3000 mg/kg/d). We have observed the following. (1) Animals can be treated with high doses of 5FC without serious toxicity. (2) Live CD+ tumors are eliminated *in vitro* by 5FC treatment. (3) Animals rejecting CD+ tumors after 5FC treatment exhibit resistance to wild type (WT) tumor. (4) Animals with preexisting disseminated WT tumor exhibit prolonged survival after treatment with CD+ tumor & 5FC. (5) IL-6 secreting tumors are rejected or grow more slowly than WT tumor. (6) Animals rejecting IL-6 secreting tumor exhibit resistance to rechallenge with WT. (7) Double transduction of tumor with CD and IL-6 allows delivery of much larger doses of cytokine secreting tumor to the host. These results suggest that live attenuated tumor vaccines can be produced with gene transfer techniques.

L-20

Antitumor Effect of Lymphokine Delivery at the Tumor Site

B. Gansbacher, E. Gilboa
Dept. of Hematologic Oncology and Molecular Biology, Memorial Sloan Kettering Cancer Center, New York, USA

Lymphokines such as IL-2 and IFN-γ are modulators of the immune response and have been used in cancer models to induce antitumor responses. These applications, however, were compromised by the short half life and toxicity of these molecules. CMS 5, a chemically induced sarcoma, is immunogenic in syngeneic hosts inducing a cellular and humoral response. We asked whether the immune response could be potentiated by the local production of IL-2 or IFN-γ by the tumor cells themself. Six recombinant N2 based retroviral vectors were constructed in which the IL-2 and the IFN-γ genes were under the control of the TK promoter, the LTR promoter and the CMV promoter respectively. CMS-5 cells were infected in vitro and G418 resistant colonies selected. Ten colonies of each infected CMS population were isolated and expanded. IL-2 and IFN-γ production was measured in a bioassay. The IL2 content in the CMS-5 supernatants ranged from 55 U/ml to 1 U/ml. IFN-γ content in the supernatants was in the range of 60 U/ml. The highest producer of each recombinant clone was used in further experiments. Southern blot and Northern blot revealed appropriate integration and mRNA production. CMS cells were then injected into groups of 5 mice. Tumor size ranged from 0–90% of the untreated control and correlated inversely with the amount of lymphokine produced. Our results demonstrate that local delivery of IL-2 and IFN-γ can result in a potent antitumor effect which correlates closely with levels of IL-2 and IFN-γ produced at the tumor site. This suggests that the way lymphokines are delivered to the tumor site can have decisive impact on the antitumor response.

L-21

Cytokine-induced Tumor Immunogenicity

F. Cavallo[a], *M. Giovarelli*[b], *A. Gulino*[b], *A. Vacca*[b], *A. Stopacciaro*[d], *A. Modesti*[c], *G. Forni*[e]
[a] University of Turin,
[b] University of L'Aquila,
[c] University of Chieti,
[d] University of La Sapienza, Rome, and
[e] Immunogenetics and Histocompatibility Center, CNR, Turin, Italy

In natural conditions, proliferating tumor cells are poorly or not at all immunogenic. Nevertheless, during the early steps of tumor recognition the presence of exogenous interleukins (ILs), as well as ILs released by IL-gene engineered tumor cells, helps the induction of an anti-tumor immune resonse. These ILs do not affect tumor proliferation. Rather, tumor inhibition is the result of their interference with control mechanisms of the immune system. In the present work, to get a realistic assessment of the immunogenic potential of cytokine releasing neoplastic cells, we used an expression vector to introduce the cDNA coding for murine IL-1, IL-2 IFN-γ, and IL-4 into the cells of a spontaneous, apparently non-immunogenic murine adenocarcinoma. On comparing the oncogenicity and immunogenicity of adenocarcinoma clones releasing different amounts of cytokines, it was found that disappearance of tumorigenicity and the acquistion of immunogenicity are connected events depending on the host immune system. The efficient induction of a tumor-specific immune memory rests on CD4 T-lymphocytes, the number transfected tumor cells used, and the amount and the combination of cytokine released. The evidence that a long-lasting tumor specific immune memory takes place following a challenge with apparently non-immunogenic adenocarcinoma cells releasing cytokines supports the notion the most tumors may become immunogenic in the presence of cytokines, and holds out the prospect of strategical employment of cytokines as a component of new tumor vaccines.

L-22 missing

L-23

Therapeutic Use of IL2 in AML. Experimental and Clinical Aspects

R. Foa, G. Meloni, A. Guarini, F. Mandelli, F. Gavosto

Dipartimento di Scienze Biomediche e Oncologia Umana, Sezione Clinica, University of Torino and Dipartimento di Biopatologia Umana, Sezione di Ematologia, University of Rome, Italy

Pre-clinical studies have demonstrated the potential feasiblity and theoretical rationale for employingt IL2/LAK cells in the management of acute leukemia patients. The clinical data so far accumulated refer mainly to the in vivo administration of IL2 alone. The results obtained indicate that IL2 may be administered to acute leukemia patients, and that the associated toxicities appear acceptable particularly using a daily dose-escalating protocol of continuous IL2 infusion. While limited effects have been observed in patients with advanced disease, complete remissions have been recorded in acute myeloid leukemias with a limited proportion of residual blasts. Some remissions have been long-lived. The administration of IL2 is followed by a marked amplification of the immune compartment of the host, documented by an increase in granular lymphocytes, expression of activation markers, enhancement of the NK and IL2-induced LAK cells, and generation of endogenous LAK effectors. These modifications occur also in bone marrow lymphocytes. Furthermore, the cycles of IL2 are coupled to the in vivo release of TNF alpha and IFN gamma. The likelihood that patients with limited disease may be a preferable target of IL2-based immunotherapy is confirmed by in vitro studies which have documented that at diagnosis and, to a further extent, at relapse leukemic blasts are most often resistant to autologous LAK effectors, whilst the killing machinery is often restored at the time of remission. The possibility of using IL2 or IL2 plus LAK cells following autografting procedures in an attempt to control/eradicate minimal residual disease has also been investigated. The rationale for such an approach is that of treating patients at a time when the tumoral burden is at its lowest peak and when LAK precursors may be found in the peripheral blood. The randomized studies currently underway will clarify the role of IL2 in acute leukemia patients.

L-24

Interleukin 2 Following Autologous Bone Marrow Transplantation or the Treatment of Malignant Solid Tumors

M. C. Favrot, S. Négrier, U. Michon, D. Blaise, R. Oskan, J. L. Bernard, P. Palmer, T. Philip

Centre Léon Berard, Lyon, France

High dose chemotherapy and autologous bone marrow transplantation (ABMT) can permit prolonged clinical remission in malignant solid tumors, but disease relapses still occur. Experimental and clinical studies have provided evidence that the use of interleukin 2 (IL2) after ABMT may prevent relapse through the stimulation of the immune system.

Various multicentric protocols have been conducted combining both therapeutic approaches, as summarized below: 1) 28 adult patients received high dose BCNU (800 mg/m^2) followed at day 3 by ABMT and day 4 by one or two cycles of 6 days continuous infusion of high dose IL2 (18 x 10^6 IU/m^2/day). Toxicity was not negligible (one toxic death) asnd one IL2 cycle appears as tolerable. In contrast, hematological recovery has not damaged. In 24 evaluable patients 4 responses were observed: One complete remission (CR) of short duration for non Hodgkin's lymphoma, one CR (30 months +) and 2 partial response (PR) (6 months) for two metastatic gastric adenocarcinomas. 2) 13 children with neuroblastoma in partial remission after induction therapy were treated with one or two courses of high use chemotherapy and ABMT, followed between day 75 and 100 post ABMT with two 5 day cycles of IL2 continuous infusion (18 x 10^6 IU/m^2/day). 12 patients are evaluable for response: 1 CR (9 months), 1 PR 9 months), 6 stable diseases and 4 progressions. Recombinant IL2 therapy did not impair hematological recover, but induced major toxicity: 2 toxic deaths and 2 early deaths (3 and 5 months) with possible causality of IL2.

The immunological follow up of both studies confirms that one or two cycles of high dose IL2 can nearly selectively increase IK-LAK cell member and functions. Results were updated in June and compared to those obtained in multicentric studies of IL2 post-ABMT in solid tumors.

L-25 missing

L-26

Transplantation of Interleukin 2 Activated Autologous Bone Marrow in Patients with Acute Myeloid Leukemia (AML)

H-G. Klingemann

Leukemia/Bone Marrow Transplantation Program of British Columbia, and Terry Fox Laboratory, Div. of Hematology, University of British Columbia, Vancouver, Canada

Relapse in AML particularly after autologous marrow grafting continues to be major problem despite the use of aggressive preparative regiments. In an attempt to induce a graft-versus-leukemia (GVL) – like mechanism, we have been exploring the possibility of culturing the marrow autograft ex vivo with interleukin 2 (IL 2) to stimulate the activation of lymphokine activated killer (LAK) cells, so that low doses of IL 2 administered immediately post-transplant might obtain an effective but non- toxic immunotherapeutic effect. In a series of preclinical experiments we were able do define culture conditions that allow the generation of strong LAK cell activity from normal or remission AML bone marrow without deleterious effects on primitive hematopoietic cells after one week at 37 °C. To assess the purging effect of such an approach, neomycin-resistant (neo^r) K562 cells were generated by electroporation of the neo^r gene so that residual leukemic cells could be uniquely detected by assaying for their ability to produce colonies in methylcellulose cultures containing G418, or by PCR for the neo^r-specific sequences. Fresh bone marrow cells from patients with AML in first remission were mixed with K562 cells (at ratios of 1 – 5 %) and then cultured with IL 2 (1000 U/ml) for 6 days. With an initial concentrations of

$\leq$ 1% K562 cells, none could be detected by PCR at the end of the 6 day period of co-culture. However, addition of > 1% K562 cells to marrow dit not result in complete eliminition of the K562 cells in all patients.
Seven patients with 'high risk' AML have now been transplanted with marrow cultured in flasks for 8 days in the presence of IL 2 (natural IL 2, Biotest Pharma, Frankfurt). All patients were conditioned with bulsulfan and cyclophosphamide and also received IL 2 s.c. at low doses from day 0 to 7 post BMT. Engraftment (WBC > 0.5 x 10^9/L) occurred between day 25 and 45. No significant adverse reactions related to the IL 2 were noted. One patient died of septicemia and ARDS. The others are alive and relapse-free at a median of 6 months post-BMT.
The results suggest the feasibility of combining leukemic cell purging and LAK cell generation maintained by subsequent IL 2 administration in vivo as a possible approach to improving effectiveness of autologous BMT for the treatment of AML.

L-27

IL-1ra Reduces the Pathology Associated with Immune Mediated Diseases but is not an Immunosuppressive Agent

Robert C. Thompson
Synergen Inc., Boulder, Co, USA

A novel inhibitor of IL-1 action that competes for the IL-1 receptor (IL-1 receptor antagonist, IL-1ra) promises to help demonstrate the role of IL-1 in animal models of human disease and in regulation of the receptor antagonist are suitable for this investigation we have established that it shows no agonist properties *in vitro* or *vivo*, and that IL-1ra interacts with the Type I and with the Type II IL-1 receptors on neutrophils and B cells. In addition we have shown that IL-1ra can block IL-1 action *in vitro* and *in vivo* when used at concentrations 100 to 1000-fold greater than that of IL-1.
IL-1ra has been tested in a number of animal models of local inflammatory disease that have some immune component. The protein reduces the intensity of joint swelling and cartilage erosion in a rat model of rheumatoid arthritis, reduces tissue necrosis and edema in a rabbit model of ulcerative colitis, and reduces bronchial hyperreactivity and granulocyte levels in a guinea pig model of asthma. Clinical trials have been initiated in all three of these disease. Preliminary results from the rheumatoid arthritis trial show a reduction in tender joints following daily treatment with IL-1a.
IL-1ra has also been tested in models of systemic inflammation and has been shown to increase survival and reduce hypotension in several models of septic shock. A Phase II trial of IL-1ra in patients with septic shock or sepsis syndrome has shown a correlation of survival with IL-1ra dosage level.
High doses of IL-1ra have no effect on the humoral or cell-mediated immune respone in mice. Although these results do not rule out a role for IL-1 in the immune system they suggest that IL-1 does not play a critical role, or that it can be replaced by other cytokines in the development of the specific immune response. However, it would appear that IL-1 has a unique role in the inflammatory response that is driven by the specific or innate immune response, or by injury.

L-28

Recombinant Human Interleukin-4 (IL-4) Given as Daily Subcutaneous Injections – a Phase I Dose Toxicity Trial

J. H. Scarffe[a], M. H. Gilleece[a], A. Gosh[c], C. M. Heyworth[b], A. P. Simmonds[d], N. Testa[b], P. Stern[c], T. M. Dexter[b]
[a] Cancer Research Campaign Depts of Medical Oncology
[b] Experimental Hematology
[c] Immunology, Christie Hospital NHS Trust, Manchester, and Schering Plough, Mildenhall, UK

Patients with a malignancy unresponsive to conventional therapy aged over 18 years who had given informed consent, were eligible for entry. It was planned for 3 patients to be entered at each for the following dose levels:.5, 1.0, 5.0, 10.0 & 25.0 μg/kg/day of IL-4 (Schering-Plough). The IL-4 was planned to be administered on days 1 (cycle 1), 8–17 (cycle 2), and 29–57 (cycle 3). There was no dose escalation within the same patient's regimen, and the study endpoint was WHO grade 3/4 toxicity in 2 out of 3 patients at that dose level.
A total of 9 patients were entered into the trial, 3 at each dose level of .5, 1.0, and 5.0 μg/kg/day. All patients completed cycle 1 and 2 of dosing and 5 patients completed all 3 cycles. Two patients at the lowest dose level withdrew from the trial because of disease progression, and 2 patients at 5.0 μg/kg/day were withdrawn at day 24 and day 32 because of WHO grade 3 toxicity. Both were pyrexial after dosing and reported severe arthralgia. Patient 8 developed hepatic encephalopathy, but analysis of stored sera revealed him to have been infected with hepatitis C at least 2 years before entry to the trial and residual liver damage may have been a factor, but his liver functions improved rapidly on stopping IL-4. Patient 9 experienced photophobia, pain in metastatic lymph nodes and vomiting. The injection of IL-4 subcutaneously was well tolerated locally with no pain or reaction at the site of injection. Generalized symptoms of toxicity such as anorexia, lethargy and flu-like symptoms occured at all dose levels, but subsided within 24 hours at the end of each cycle. Dose increments were associated with symptoms of increasing severity.
Modest dose related increases in peripheral blood neutrophil and platelet counts were observed. No significant changes in bone marrow morphology or number of progenitor cells were seen. No consistent or significant changes were observed in a wide range of immunological testing. There was no evidence of responses although one patient with myeloma had a transient fall in his paraprotein. 1 μg/kg/day subcutaneously is a relatively well tolerated dose of IL-4 to take forward into Phase II trials.

L-29

Biological Properties of Human IL-10

R. de Waal Malefyt, J. E. de Vries
DNAX Research Institute, Palo Alto, CA, USA

Despite its history, evidence is accumulating that IL-10 plays a major role in suppressing immune- and inflammatory responses. IL-10 is produced by many cell types, including human Th0, Th1 and Th2 T cell clones, B cells and monocytes. IL-10 prevents antigen specific T cell proliferation which is associated with downregulation of class II MHC expression on antigen-presenting monocytes. IL-10 inhibits not only the proliferation of human T cell clones towards protein antigens, but also to alloantigens. In additon, IL-10 inhibits proliferation and cytotoxicity generated in primary mixed leukocyte cultures. IL-10 inhibits cytokine production by PBMNC, T cell clones, monocytes and NK cells. IL-10 specifically inhibits the production of IL-2 by T cell clones, IL-10 strongly blocks the production of the proinflammatory cytokines IL-1α, IL-1β, IL-6, IL-8 and TNFα by monocytes whereas it upregulates the production of IL-1RA by these cells. IL-10 inhibits also the IL-2 induced production of IFN-γ and TNFα by NK cells. However it enhances the IL-2 induced LAK activity. Thus, IL-10 suppresses immune and inflammatory responses and could play a role in tolerance following bone marrow or organ transplantation. The present knowledge of the structure and function of IL-10 and its possible role in cancer will be discussed.

L-30

Regulatory Effects of TGFβ on the Immune System and Tumor Cell Growth[1]

J. Kekow, W.L. Gross

Dept. of Clinical Rheumatology, Medical University of Lübeck, and Dept. of Medicine, Rheumaklinik Bad Bramstedt

Current interest in clinical research of transforming growth factor β (TGFβ) results from its multiple actions on almost every cell type and the potential therapeutic use. The bioactive protein, a 25KDa homodimer, exists in man mostly in the TGFβ1 isoform. The pleiotropic character is shown by the stimulatory effect on mesenchymal cells while proliferation of other cells, e.g. epithelial cells and lymphocytes, is suppressed. The influence on the immune system is, however, not restricted to global anti-proliferating effects. Concering T-cell proliferation, we could observe a preferential inhibition of CD4 positive T-cells. This may contribute, at least in part, to the depletion of CD4 positive cells in AIDS, as this retroviral disease shows TGFβ overexpression quite similar to adult T-cell leukemia. In addition, TGFβ suppresses both B-cell proliferation and differentiation. This may explain defects of the humoral immune response even in hypergammaglobulinemia, also typical for HIV infection and systemic autoimmune diseases. Further important modulating effects on the immune system consist in suppression of cytotoxic T-cells, LAK-cells, and NK-cells. TGFβ downregulates HLA-DR expression and production of many proinflammatory cytokines (e.g. TNFα, IL1). in oncology, research indicates that the development of epithelial cell tumors may be partially due to an escape from autocrine of paracrine growth control by TGFβ. This can involve a loss of TGFβ receptors on the tumor cells, and may be induced by a failure in the intracellular growth control pathway mediated by TGFβ. Interestingly, B-cells infected with EBV, escape also from TGFβ growth control and start to proliferate, which can explain the high incidence of B-cell lymphomas in AIDS. Further clinical excitement comes from the observation, that artificial TGFβ overexpression in fibrosarcoma results in a loss of tumor defense mechanisms. Taken together, TGFβ represents a strong immunomodular capable to influence directly or indirectly (tumor) cell growth. Further studies have to show possible clinical applications. Some promising data are already given by the clinical benefit of tamoxifen and retinoids in selected malignancies, agents inducing TGFβ.

[1] Supported by a grant from the BMFT FKZ 01 VM 8906/8, and the BMFT program 'Autoimmunity'

L-31

Involvement of Cytokines in GVHD and GVL

E. Holler, H.J. Kolb, J. Mittermüller, S. Thierfelder, W. Wilmanns

Medizin. Klinik III, Klin. Großhadern, Inst. f. Klinische Hämatologie und Immunologie der GSF, Munich

Allogeneic bone marrow transplantation (BMT) results in complex immune interactions between donor immunocompetent cells and recipient tissues. While acute graft-vs.-host disease (aGvHd) is a major cause of transplant related morbidity and mortality, there is increasing evidence that immunologic control of residual malignant cells by graft-vs-leukemia effects (GvL) is a major therapeutic principle of BMT. Attempts to reduce GvHD by removal of donor T cells resulted in an increased incidence of relapse demonstrating the close association of GvHD and GvL mechanisms. Consideration of cytokine interactions might allow more differentiated manipulation of GvHD and GvL. Recent studies suggest that aGvHD is far more a 'cytokine disease' than a syndrome mediated by cellular effectors. We and others were able to demonstrate a central role of TNFα (and IL6) released by recipient cells in induction of early tissue damage and aGvHD following BMT. In addition, TNFα and IFN-gamma released by donor T helper cells are central effectors in aGvHD. Experimental as well as first clinical data indicate sufficient efficacy of anti-cytokine strategies as new modalities for treatment and prophylaxis of aGvHD.
However, the role of these cytokines as effectors exerting GvL as well as the cells and the targets involved in GvL are still poorly defined though there are reports on induction of GvL in the absence of GvHD by infusion of donor lymphocytes or IL2. In summary, careful further studies are needed to answer if cytokine modulation will allow separation of GvHD and GvL in the future.

L-32

Cytokine Induced Adhesion Molecules and Tumor Spread

R. Giavazzi, A. Garofalo, I. Martin-Padura, E. Dejana

Mario Negri Institute for Pharmacological Research Bergamo and Milano, Italy

A major target of inflammatory stimuli is the vascular endothelium which responds with specific morphological and metabolic changes. The cytokines IL-1 and TNF induce the synthesis or augmented expression of edhesion molecules on endothelial cells causing increased adhesiveness for different subsets of leukocytes. Similarly the adhesion of human tumor cells is augmented on cultured endothelial cells activated by IL-1 and TNF. Adhesion studies in the presence of monoclonal antibodies that selectively recognize adhesive molecules on endothelial cells or their ligands on tumor cells indicate the attachment of tumor cells to cytokine-activated endothelial cells is mediated by specific recognitioni mechanisms. IL-1 given to mice before the i.v. injection of tumor cells (experimental metastasis) or during primary tumor growth and metastatization (spontaneous metastasis) resulted in the augmentation of lung metastases, without significant effect on the primary tumor growth. In addition IL-1 given to mice before intravenous injection of radiolabelled tumor cells augmented their retention in the lung, thus indicating the increase in metastases induced by IL-1, in vivo, might be associated to endothelial cell activation/tumor cell adhesion described in vitro. The role of adhesion molecules in tumor spread and metastasis formation, in vivo, will be addressed.

Free Communications (Part I)

T-1

Vinblastine (VLB) with/without Natural Human Fibroblast Interferon (HuIFN)-β) in Metastatic Renal Cell Carcinoma (RCC)

E. A. Abdi, P. M. Venner, S. Bishop, Y. H. Tan, T. A. McPherson
Cross Cancer Institute, Edmonton, Canada

Few clinical trials in cancer have been conducted using HuIFN-β. Thirty-two consecutive patients with previously untreated metastatic RCC were treated with VLB (.2 mg / kg) every 3 weeks (n=15; 10 males, 5 females) or same dose and frequency of VLB combined with HuIFN-β (30 MU / m^2 / d) for 4 consecutive days each week continuously (n=17; 13 males, 4 females). The median ages for HuIFN-β +VLB or VLB alone patients were 58.5 (42-83) and 58.3 (36-80) years respectively. 15 patients allocated HuIFN-β +VLB but 6 allocated VLB had prior nephrectomy at a median of 15.3 and 11.5 months respectivelly. A median of 5.5 (1-11) cycles of HuIFN-β +VLB and 5.4 (1-13) cycles of VLB alone were given. Of 17 patients on HuIFN-β +VLB arm, 6 (2 CR, 4 PR) responded, 5 had stable disease (SD), 4 had progression (PD). Of 15 patients on VLB arm, 3 (all PR) responded, 9 had SD (including 2 mixed responses), 3 had PD. One patient on each of the treatment arms was unassessable due to treatment toxicity. Reversible Grade 4 thrombocytopenia was seen in 1 patient on each of the two arms. One patient on HuIFN-β developed ITP and another developed pulmonary sarcoidosis due to IFN. Average weight loss of 7.3% on HuIFN-β and 3.4% on VLB alone was observed. Flu-like symptoms were observed in the majority of patients while on HuIFN-β but were manageable with the regular use of acetaminophen +/- prednisone and the development of tachyphylaxis. No hepatic, renal, cardiac or pulmonary toxicity was observed. Peripheral neuropathy was seen with equal frequency in the two arms. No psychiatric toxicity was seen. One patient achieving CR to HuIFN-β died from an intracerebral hemorrhage from a microscopic focus of metastatic RCC. NK-cell activity increased during the first 2-3 cycles of HuIFN-β but then achieved a plateau. No correlation between anti-tumor activity and changes in NK-cell, lymphocyte or monocyte count was observed. No anti-IFN antibody was seen. The median survival for HuIFN-β +VLB patients was 21 months but 7 months for VLB patients (ns). Seven patients on HuIFN-β +VLB arm and 5 patients on VLB arm are alive with/without disease at a median of 22.9 and 16.2 months, respectively. Survival of all responders (CR, PR and SD) was 21 vs. 3 months for PD (p=.009). Due to small patient numbers, more detailed analysis of survival based on response achieved with each treatment cannot be performed. The effect of prior nephrectomy on survival cannot be assessed.
Our combination of HuIFN-β +VLB has manageable toxicity and appears to have more anti-tumor activity than VLB alone however due to small sample size no statistically significant survival advantage has been demonstrated.

T-2

Biomodulatory Priming of Melanoma Metastasis: Rationale and Feasibility

H. Voigt, R. Claßen, J. Ramaker
Melanoma Research Project, Kaltenkirchen/Holstein

Introduction: In order to improve the palliative outcome in metastatic malignant melanoma various attempts have been made to introduce cytotoxic drug combinations or those combining biomodulatory together with anti-neoplastic agents. However, most therapeutic regimens yielded disappointingly low responses of short duration with reasonable toxicity. In this respect, one of the major obstacles considered in melanoma therapy is the fact that primary or secondary drug resistance phenomena are likely to interfere with the drug schedules used, and that the overall state of knowledge of the biomodulatory mode of action, the pharmacodynamic properties, and the varying drug interactions is still marginal. Therefore, a phase-oriented investigative protocol has been delineated combining targeted biomodulation, tamoxifen-induced reversal of multidrug resistance (MDR), and cytotoxic action in order to improve primary response rates as well as response duration in metastatic disease.
Methods: The protocol applied consisted of Interferon α-2b (rIFN-α-2b) I.L. / P.L. 3-5 Mio IU D1-D7, 10 Mio IU D8-D14 together with tamoxifen-HD (TAM) 160 MG P.O., BCNU 150 MG/BSA I.V. D15, CDDP 25 MG/BSA I.V. D15-D17, and DTIC 220 MG/BSA I.V. D15-D17. Treatment cycles were repeated monthly with BCNU given every second cycle until disease progression.
Results: Serial evaluation of lab parameters (weekly), tamoxifen concentrations (plasma and tissue), punch biopsy histology, and analysis of clinical and radiographic tumor dimensions (biweekly) indicate that the ITBCD-protocol is capable of inducing effective biomodulatory priming of the target tissues thus preparing metastatic tumor sites for amplified cytotoxic action. Toxicity of the regimen employed was mainly hematologic consisting of neutropenia/thrombocytopenia from the second cycle onwards, but requiring dosage modification only for interferon. Responses were found in all of the patients treated so far with 1 CR, 1 PR, and 2 MR among four initially treated patients. In the latter two patients extensive cytoreductive surgery became feasible subsequently leading to NED-status.
Conclusion: Although final conclusions can not yet be drawn from the preliminary results in this ongoing study, the protocol described offers amplified presuppositions for inducing improved tumor regressions in far advanced tumor stages. Prospective trial data will still be needed to confirm the preliminary experiences reported, particularly in view of the optimal time schedule and sequencing of modalities.

T-3

Differentiation Therapy with Interferon α plus Low-dose Cytarabine in Acute Monoblastic Leukemia Patients

H. T. Hassan[a, b], *H. R. Maurer*[b]
[a] Department of Hematology, Medical Research Institute, University of Alexandria, Egypt
[b] Institut für Pharmazie, Freie Universität Berlin

As acute monoblastic leukemia (AMoL) is a malignant disease in which neither conventional intensive chemotherapy nor BMT was beneficial, it is justified in this disease to evaluate the efficacy of Interferon α (IFN-α) that seems promising on the basis of a possible role for its juxtapositioned genes in the pathogenesis of the differentiation defect in some AMoL patients, of its regulatory effect in monocyte differentiation and of its success in the treatment of chronic leukemias. Six children with untreated primary AMoL (their median age was 9.8 years; range, 7.5 - 13) were treated with recombinant human IFN-α (3 million Units / m^2 / day subcutaneously three times weekly) plus low-dose cytarabine (10 mg / m^2 / day subcutaneously daily) for 21 days with or without hydroxyurea (HU) (50 mg / kg / day orally daily only for patients with WBC counts of $\geq 50 \times 10^9/l$) for 10 days in a clinical pilot study. Prophylactic paracetamol, antibiotics and allopurine were given orally daily to suppress concomitant influenzal symptoms, fever and prevent infections and urate nephropathy. After two treatment courses, 4 patients achieved complete remission and 2 had partial remission. Also, HU was effective in reducing the leukemic mass and preventing leukostasis in the patients with WBC count of $\geq 50 \times 10^9/l$. Therapy was well tolerated, with thrombocytopenia comprising the prominant side effect which required frequent platelet transfusions (median: 4 units per treatment course, range: 2 - 7). Upon the achievement of complete remission, CNS prophylaxis with cranial irradiation was administered followed by maintenance therapy with 6-thioguanine plus hydroxyurea for 7 days every three weeks. For follow-up durations of ten months or more, the four patients have sustained ongoing complete remission. Both IFN-α and low-dose cytarabine induced in vitro differentiation of human acute monoblastic leukemia cells. These promising results warrant confirmation and randomised comparison with established regimens to determine any survival advantage in large clinical studies for leukemia patients aged ≥ 6 years.

T-4

Intraperitoneal (IP) Administration of Tumor Necrosis Factor (rTNF) in Combination with Interferon α (rIFN) or γ (rIFN) in 22 Patients with Tumor Persistence of Ovarian Cancer (OC). A Phase II Study

M. Kaufmann[a], *H. Schmid*[a], *E. M. Grischke*[a], *G. Minckwitz*[a], *G. Bastert*[a], *J. Kempin*[c], *U. Raeth*[b]

[a] Univ.-Frauenklinik und

[b] Med.-Univ.-Klinik Heidelberg

[c] Knoll AG Ludwigshafen

TNF shows pleiotropic effects, probably all promoting its anti-tumor action. In vitro and in animals bearing TNF sensitive tumors TNF is one of the most active anti-tumor agents. However, its therapeutic index seems to be very narrow despite of advances in supportive treatment (e. g. with paracetamol, indomethacin, pethidine). Therefore synergistic combinations are warranted (e. g. with IFNα, IFNγ, cytotoxics as cisplatin. adriamycin, cytoxan) or a breakthrough of TNF resistance should be aimed (e. g. by time-optimized application of other cytokins). Our group has already shown the efficacy of rTNF IP administration for malignant ascites control in patients with ovarian, breast, GI or other tumors. The overall response rate in 71 patients was 77%, the dosage of rTNF was .08 - .14 mg / m^2 IP weekly, median 2.5 applications. Solid tumor mass was not affected. rIFNα was IP applicated (<30^6 U / m^2 single dose, max. 6x) in 9 patients with OC with microscopic (R1) or minimal macroscopic (R2: <.5 cm) residual tumor after second look operation (SLOP) or laparascopy (LSCOP). Again no measurable effect on solid tumor was seen. All 9 patients relapsed.

Therefore, in 22 heavily pretreated patients with OC after SLOP / LSCOP we used a combination of rTNF (.14 mg / m^2) IP and 6 hours later rIFNα (20^6 U / m^2) IP every second week, 6 x (n=8) or rTNF(dosis-escalated from .04, .08 to .14 mg / m^2) IP and 2 to 6 hours later rIFNγ (dosis escalated from .04, .08 to .14 mg/m^2) IP weekly, 4 x (n=14). Median age was 51 (28 - 64) years, WHO-performance status 0 - 2.

Results of IFNα: 2 of 8 patients with minimal macroscopic tumor <.2 cm showed no progression after 15, resp. 18 months. 2 of 8 patients with minimal macroscopic tumor <.5 cm had a progression after 3 and 9 months. In 4 of 8 patients with macroscopic tumor >.5 cm no measurable response was seen, however ascites was disolved.

Results of IFNα: In 4 of 14 patients with lower dosis of IFNα (.04, respectively .08 mg / m^2) there was only 1 partial response in ascites control, 3 compartimentation and no effect on solid tumor. In 10 of 14 patients (.14 mg / m^2 IFNγ) 2 complete remissions of ascites and minimal macroscopic tumor <.2 cm could be reached, in 1 case histologically proven. These 2 patients had no progression after 28 and 30 months. 8 of these 10 patients showed response in ascites control, but no measurable effect on macroscopic tumor >.2 cm. In all 22 patients side effects were tolerable (no WHO-grade III / IV) by prophylactic supportive therapy with indomethacin.

Conclusions: Cytokin combination therapies of TNF IP and IFN IP or IFNγ IP are effective means in ascites control of OC. In contrast to mono-cytokin-IP-therapies with TNF or IFNα, the combined therapy showed response in solid tumors. Yet it was only seen in patients with minimal tumor burdon <.2 cm. The dosis-escalated IFNγ study is still ongoing. For solid tumors >.2 cm new combination therapies are warranted. Side effects were tolerable due to supportive therapy.

T-5

Low-dose IL-2 and IFN-β Modulate IFN-γ Synthesis in Hairy-cell Leukemia Patients

A. M. Liberati[a], *S. Mancini*[a], *D. Adiuto*[b], *M. Cecchini*[a], *M. Schippa*[a], *V. De Angelis*[a], *L. Fedeli*[b], *R. Palumbo*[b], *F. Grignani*[a]

[a] Istituto Clinica Medica Ia, Universita di Perugia

[b] Servizio di Medicina Nucleare, Policlinico Monteluce Perugia, Italy

Active phase disease hairy-cell leukemia (HCL) patients have a defect in in vitro production of PHA-induced IFN-γ. The defect tends to decrease and then disappears in patients treated with IFN-β who achieve complete or partial clinical-hematological and histological remission. Significant quantities of IFN-γ (Centocor Diagnostics), but not IL-2 (Ami-Advanced Magnetic, Inc.), have been found in supernatants of mononucleated cell samples obtained from HCL patients treated in vivo with combined IL-2 / IFN-β (5 IU / ml + 10 IU / ml), but not PHA. The concentration of IFN-γ was much greater in IL-2 / IFN-β treated samples from patient in the active phase of the disease than in untreated cultures in 5 / 10 experiments, as well as in 13 / 24 samples from patients in remission. The mean IFN-γ level ±SE in 10 treated cultures from active phase patients was 8±3.6 (versus means .7±SE .4 untreated preparations) and 24±6.1 in those from in remission patients (versus means 3±SE 2.1 in controls). Inrespective of the phase of the disease, IFN-γ production was higher in cultures treated with IL-2 / IFN-β that also displayed increased cytolytic activity against the K562 line (means IFN-γ levels $\pm$SE 21.9$\pm$5 versus 2.4$\pm$1.7 in controls). In contrast, in those cultures where the IL-2 / IFN-β combinations failed to stimulate cytolytic activity versus the K562 line, the levels of IFN-γ was not significantly higher than in untreated controls (1.9$\pm$.5 versus 1.1$\pm$.7). It would therefore seem that, when added together, low-doses of IL-2 and IFN-β are able to induce IFN-γ production and stimulate NK-cell activity in PBMC obtained from HCL patients.

T-6

Inhibition of Erythropoietin Production by the Monokines IL-1 and TNF-α

W. Jelkmann, J. Fandrey, H. Pagel
Dept. of Physiology, University of Bonn

The blood level of erythropoietin (Epo) is often inappropriately low for the degree of anemia in patients with infectious, inflammatory or malignant diseases. To investigate the nature of this deficiency we studied the effects of macrophage-conditioned media and of various pure recombinant human cytokines on the production of Epo in human hepatoma cultures of the line HepG2. In addition, some of the cytokines were tested for their effect on hypoxia-induced Epo synthesis in isolated perfused rat kidneys.
Hypoxic HepG2 cultures were measured to produce about .3 IU Epo per mg cell protein and 24 hours. This basal rate of the production of Epo was significantly lowered when conditioned medium from LPS-stimulated mouse macrophages was added to HepG2-cells or when these were co-cultured with LPS-stimulated rat kidney mesangiocytes. The addition of pure Interleukin (IL)-1β, IL-1α, or tumor necrosis factor α (TNF-α) also resulted in a dose-dependent decrease of Epo production, with half-maximal inhibition at 2,5 and 200 U / ml, respectively. IL-6, transforming growth factor β, and Interferon γ did not inhibit. In addition, IL-1β and TNF-α were shown to suppress Epo synthesis in isolated rat kidneys perfused with hypoxic medium for 3 hours.
Our findings provide evidence that inflammatory monokines may play a role in the pathogenesis of Epo deficiency in diseases associated with immune reactions.

T-7

Biological Activity of Mutants of Human Tumor Necrosis Factor

R. Kircheis[a], J. Milleck[a], V. G. Korobko[b], L. N. Shingarova[b], D. Behnke[c], H. E. Schmidt[a]
[a] Max-Delbrück-Center for Molecular Medicine, Berlin-Buch
[b] Inst. for Bioorganic Chemistry, Acad. of Sci. Moscow, Russia
[c] Inst. for Microbiol. Exper. Therapy, Jena

Point mutations in different regions of the hTNF-α molecule have been shown to influence its cytotoxic and cytostatic activity as well as the extend of hemorrhagic tumour necrosis and lethal toxicity in mice. Double mutation in positions 150 and 155 of the C-terminal region decreased the cytotoxicity on murine L929 fibroblasts and human MCF-7 mammary carcinoma cells. Competitive binding experiments with ^{125}J-labeled hTNF-α revealed that the loss of cytotoxicity was caused by a loss of binding to the target cells. In contrast to the reduced activity of the hTNF-α mutant towards L929 and MCF-7-cells neither its binding nor its cytostatic activity on the human myeloic leukemia cell lines HL60 and U937 were affected. These target cell dependent effects make it likely that the L929 and MCF-7-cells express a different type of TNF-α receptor than the myeloic leukemia cells.
A mutation in position 127 decreased the overall activity of hTNF-α while a deletion of the 4 N-terminal amino-acids did not reduce its biological activity.
With regard to in vivo experiments the hTNF-α mutants differed in their anti-tumour effects and lethal toxicity. A segregation of the anti-tumour activity on the one hand and toxicity on the other has, however, not been observed.

T-8

Regulation of H_4Biopterin Synthesis in Human Mononuclear Cells during Immune Response

I. Ziegler, K. Schott, M. Gütlich
GSF-Institut für Klinische Molekularbiologie und Tumorgenetik, München

In addition to its established cofactor function, H_4biopterin has more recently been shown to increase the affinity of the IL-2 receptor to its ligand and to affect various aspects of T-cell proliferation (for review see Ziegler I: Med Res Rev 1990;10:95). A transient biosynthesis of this modulator occurs during lectin stimulation of resting T-cells. Furthermore, IFN-γ induces neopterin synthesis in monocytes/macrophages (Huber C, et al: J Exp Med 1984;160:310.). In cooperation with IL-2, it causes a transient H_4biopterin accumulation in primed T-cells. The time courses could satisfactorily be explained by the specific activities of the relevant enzymes (Ziegler I, et al: J Biol Chem 1990;265:17045). In particular, they correlate with the activity of GTP-cyclohydrolase I (GTP-CH), the initial enzyme of H_4biopterin synthesis. The regulation level of this enzyme however, remained unknown. We have now constructed a 555 bp cDNA probe specific for human GTP-CH mRNA. We demonstrate that in each case the upregulation of GTP-CH activity correlates with increased steady state mRNA levels. In addition, the enhancement of IFN-γ induced enzyme activity in activated T-cells by IL-2 corresponds to further increases in mRNA expression. However, mRNA levels remain stable despite a steep decline in enzyme activity following the culmination. This indicates that the rapidly progressing down-regulation of the activity is caused by post-translational modification of the protein, probably by dephosphorylation. In summary, the data provide evidence for a stringent control of H_4biopterin synthesis in the immune network by coordination of translational and post-translational regulation of GTP-CH.

T-9

r-GM-CSF Augments rHu-IL-4 Induced ADCC of Human Peripheral Blood Mononuclear Cells in Presence of MAb 17-1A

G. Masucci, E. Reali, H. Mellstedt
Dept. of Oncology, Radiumhemmet, Karolinska Hospital, Stockholm, Sweden

In animal and in vitro experimental systems, antibody-dependent cellular cytotoxicity (ADCC) has been claimed to be an important mechanism for tumor cell destruction mediated by monoclonal antibodies (MAbs). In vitro, the main mononuclear cell subpopulation responsible for ADCC are NK/K-cells and monocytes/macrophages. We have previously demonstrated IL-4 and GM-CSF (Schering-Plough Co., USA) increased monocytes and NK/K-cells ADCC mediated by MAb17-1A (Centocor, USA) recognizing a tumor associated antigen, CO17-1A, present on colon cancer cell line SW948. A possible scenario in the future tumor immunotherapy might be combination of various biologic agents with different activities on the immune system. In this study we investigate whether the ADCC could be further enhanced by activating effector cells with GM-CSF and IL-4 at different concentrations and temporal sequences. Human PBMC were treated sequentially either by GM-CSF for 1, 2, 4 hours first and IL-4 thereafter or vice versa. The effect of these cytokines on PBMC cytolytic activity was measured on a 18 hours ADCC assay mediated by MAb17-1A (mouse IgG2a) against the colon cancer cell line SW1116. We found a priming with GM-CSF at optimal concentration ($10^{-3}\mu g/ml$) for 1, 2, 4 hours significantly enhanced the following IL-4 induced activation of PBMC. GM-CSF increased IL-4 generated cytotoxicity also at suboptimal concentration ($10^{-4}\mu g/ml$) after 2 hours of incubation. On the contrary a first exposure to IL-4 at optimal or suboptimal concentrations followed by GM-CSF did not show any further increase of ADCC. The expression in number and intensity of Fc receptors (I, II, III) did not follow the enhancement of cytotoxicity induced by cytokines. These findings suggest that in clinical situations, it might be important to find, first in vitro, the most efficacious combinations of different biological therapeutics achieving, then, the right sequence with antitumoral effect for in vivo delivery.

T-10

Immunotherapy and Chemotherapy in Anaplastic Thyroid Carcinoma – an Experimental Study

H. J. C. Wenisch, B. Müller, L. Bergmann, H. P. Fortmeyer, A. Encke
Dept. of Surgery, Johann-Wolfgang-Goethe-University, Frankfurt am Main

Prognosis of human anaplastic thyroid carcinoma is very poor. Recently, an increase of survival times was reported by several groups using a combination of surgery, chemotherapy, and irradiation. We could demonstrate in earlier studies, that the nude mouse-xenotransplantation model can be used for tests of several chemotherapeutic regimens. Aim of the following study was to investigate the influence of chemotherapy and/or Interferon α-2b.

Material and Methods: Four groups of each 20 nude mice (NMRI-nu/nu) were used. Slices of a originally human anaplastic thyroid carcinoma serially passaged before were grafted subcutaneously. 18 days after, therapy was started. 18 days later, the animals were sacrificed after i. v. application of 5-bromodesoxiuridine. The grafts were weighted and prepared for histological investigations. Animals of group I received doxorubicin in a dosage of 3.25 mg/kg b. w. i. v. once a week. Animals of group II received the same weekly dose of doxorubicine, and additionally 10.000 IU of Interferon α s. c. three times a week. The third group was treated with Interferon α-2b only, and the controls received isotonic saline.

Results: During therapy, statistically significant size differences developed in all of the therapy groups compared to the controls. The weight of the grafts was statistically significant lower in animals treated with Interferon α-2b. The lowest tumor weights were observed using the combination of doxorubicin and Interferon α-2b. The adverse effect on tumor proliferation was significantly less, when doxorubicin was given alone. The data of the histological studies counting the number of cells positive for 5-bromodesoxiuridine corresponded with the growth reducing effect.

Conclusions: Using the nude mouse xenotransplantation model, a growth reducting effect could be demonstrated by chemotherapy with doxorubicin. This effect was enhanced by combination with Interferon α-2b. Even after monotherapy with Interferon α-2b, a statistically significant growth inhibition was observed. Further studies must show, if comparable data can be obtained in different anaplastic thyroid carcinomas, and if a combination of Interferon α-2b and chemotherapy is able to improve the results of clinical treatment of patients with anaplastic thyroid carcinomas.

Free Communications (Part II)

F-1

Immune Functions and Clinical Response in Renal Cell Cancer Patients Receiving low-doses Cyclophosphamide, Interleukin-2 and Interferon-α

J. P. Wersäll, G. Masucci, H. Mellstedt
Dept. of Oncology (Radiumhemmet), Karolinska Hospital, Stockholm, Sweden

Pretreatment with cyclophosphamide (CY), has been claimed to inhibit suppressor functions and increase the immunomodulatory effects of IL-2. We investigated the combined treatment with low-doses CY, Interferon-α (IFN-α) and continuous infusions of IL-2 (Proleukin®, Eurocetus) in patients with renal cancer (stadium IV). 16 patients received 4 cycles of CY (500 mg/m^2) and daily injections of IFN-α 3×10^6 IU i. m. and continuous infusions of 18×10^6 IU r-IL-2 days 4–9). The cycle interval was 3 weeks. The patients were followed regularly by peripheral blood differential cell counts and serum IL-2 concentrations. We observed 3 PR (+7, +14, +12 months), 5 SD (+14, +10, +8, +6, +5 months). 8 patients progressed. No patient required intensive care. Side effects were mainly fever, malaise, capillary leak syndrome and diarrhea. Lymphocytes and neutrophils were significantly higher in responders while non responders had significantly higher eosinphils and monocytes. Serum IL-2 concentrations correlated positively to response and closely paralleled serum creatinine levels. Various immune functions were analyzed. CD 25+ cells increased significantly in all patients showing a response and correlated with the changes in $CD3^+/CD56^-$ cells. $CD3^-/CD56^+$ cells increased, while $CD29^+$ and $CD45R^+$, $CD11c^+$ and $CD54^+$ cells decreased in responders after treatment. Spontaneous cytotoxicity against NK insensitive A 498, renal cell cancer cell line was undetectable in non-responders but increased significantly and was positively related to the change in percentage of $CD3^-/CD56^+$ cells in responders. In 3 responders, Ti-γ/δ^+ cells increased significantly; these developed at the same time a thyroid gland dysfunction.

F-2

Vaccination with Modified Autologous Tumor Material and rIL-2 / rIFN-α for Treatment of Advanced Renal Cell Carcinoma

S. Pomer, R. Thiele, V. Schirrmacher, G. Staehler
Dept. of Urology, Univ. of Heidelberg, Germany

40 patients with advanced renal cell carcinoma (RCC) were entered after nephrectomy into a protocol consisting of vaccination with modified autologous tumor material and subsequent repetitive weekly cycles of Interleukin-2 (IL-2) and Interferon-α-2 b (IFN-α-2 b) at a lower subcutaneous dose (9.0_2 million IU / m^2 every 12 hours on 2 days and 5 million IU / m^2, once a day on days 1, 3 and 5, resp. The inpatient treatment was followed by a 6-week maintenance phase during which 1.8 million IU / m^2 IL-2 was given subcutaneously every 12 hours on days 1 - 5 and IFN 5 million IU / m^2 on days one, three and five administered on an outpatient basis.

All patients completed the induction week and 3 months of home therapy. No grade 3 and 4 toxicities occurred during the therapy and not a single patient had the therapy discontinued at this stage because of toxicity due to IL-2 or IFN. Of the 40 evaluable RCC patients, 5 had a complete response and 6 had partial remissions.

In further course of treatment clinical deterioration was the reason for stopping the therapy in 18 remarkably slowly progressing patients.

We conclude that the vaccination with autologous tumor material combined with subcutaneous IL-2 and IFN administration on a long term outpatient basis can induce regressions in patients with advanced RCC and even in non-responding patients a more stable course of disease can be obtained.

F-3

Inhalation of Natural Interleukin-2: Effectivity and Toxicity in Patients with Pulmonary Metastases of Renal Cell Carcinoma

E. Huland, H. Heinzer, H. Schwaibold, H. Huland
Dept. of Urology, University Clinic Eppendorf

We have been the first group to show that inhalative Interleukin-2 (IL-2) application combined with systematic i. v. IL-2 and s. c. IFN-α has low toxicity but is highly effective (J Urol, February 1992). However, cyclic inpatient i. v. application of IL-2 contributed - almost exclusively - to toxicity grade II and its therapeutic value was not clear. We report on a complete outpatient schedule in 15 patients with pulmonary metastases of renal cell carcinoma (RCC) based on 5 times daily inhalation of IL-2 (5x200,000 IU), one daily low-dose s. c. injection of IL-2 (100,000 IU / day) (90% of total IL-2 dose was given per inhalation) and 3 x / week s. c. IFN-α (15 million IU / week). Median treatment duration was 10 months (1 - 21 m). Toxicity was low, no fever, no vascular leakage, only grade I toxicity WHO, except for one grade II event. Pulmonary response reached 100%: I complete response (6.7%), 8 partial responses (53.6%), 6 cases of stable disease (40.2%), no progression during treatment. 4 of 15 patients responded with non-pulmonary metastases (3 PR, 1 SD). Patient survival is increased significantly (expected median survival 8 months, actual survival 15.3 months, 12 of 15 patients are alive. Inhalative Interleukin-2 application offers the most effective and non-toxic new approach to pulmonary metastases of RCC, achieving dramatic response rates and improving patients quality of life and life expectancy.

F-4

Antibody Formation to Interleukin-2 in Patients Treated by Aerosol Therapy: Comparison of ELISA- and Western Blot Data

U. Schwuléra[a], E. Huland[b], W. Struff[a], R. Lissner[a]
[a] Biotest Pharma GmbH, Dreieich
[b] Dept. of Urology, Klinikum Eppendorf, Hamburg

So far no information is available whether local administration of Interleukin-2, administrated via inhalation leads to an antibody response or not. 14 unselected patients with metastatic renal cell carcinoma were treated with natural Interleukin-2 (nIL-2, Biotest) and 5 patients with recombinant IL-2 expressed in E. coli (rIL-2). Details of the therapy protocol are given in the abstract of E. Huland et al. Immunoblot techniques, an ELISA and neutralization of biologic activity were used to detect and characterize specific IgG and IgM antibodies in human sera. Our data clearly indicated that all rIL-2 treated patients form antibodies with differents titers against the non-glycosylated form of IL-2, while only one patient treated with nIL-2 developed anti-IL-2 antibodies. The ELISA data were confirmed by the western blot results. This response in respect to rIL-2 occurs in the first weeks of treatment. The antibodies are mainly of the IgG subclass. Only some patients show a neutralizing activity which possibly could impair clinical efficacy.

These data clearly show that the antigenity of E. coli expressed non-glycosylated IL-2 is clearly stronger and different from glycosylated IL-2 molecules.

F-5

Lysis of Pulmonary Fibroblasts by Lymphokine (IL-2) Activated Killer Cells

R. Zambello, L. Trentin, P. Bulian, C. Agostini, A. Cipriani, G. Semenzato
Padua University School of Medicine, Dept. of Clinical Medicine, 1st Medical Clinic and Clinical Immunology Branch; Dept. of Pneumothysiology of Padua Hospital, Padua, Italy

Adoptive immunotherapy using lymphokine (IL-2) activated killer (LAK) cells has recently triggered great interest in immunologists and oncohematologists because of its therapeutic possibilities in the treatment of cancer. LAK-cells, without previous sensitization, show a wide spectrum of cytotoxicity which encompasses natural killer (NK) sensitive, NK resistant targets, and cell lines obtained from fresh or cryopreserved autologous and/or allogeneic tumors. In contrast, it is thought that LAK-cells spare the normal counterpart. Although promising clinical responses have been observed with LAK-cell therapy by different groups, a series of adverse reactions has been reported to be associated with this therapy. In particular, recently published papers pointed out the putative toxicity of LAK-cells against normal cells, including endothelial cells, monocytic/macrophage cells and keratinocytes.

In this study we addressed the question of whether LAK-cells may bind and exert lytic activity against non-transformed fibroblasts obtained from the lung. We demonstrated that human LAK-cells generated in vitro following incubation of peripheral blood mononuclear cells (PBL-LAK) or lymphocytes obtained from bronchoalveolar lavage (BAL-LAK) with recombinant IL-2 were able to bind and lyse normal lung fibroblasts obtained from transbronchial lung biopsies in a 4 hour ^{51}Cr release assay.

Both autologous and allogeneic fibroblasts were consistently bound and lysed by LAK-cells, thus suggesting that the phenomenon we observed does not require Major Histocompatibility Complex restriction. Preincubation of fibroblasts with different cytokines (IL-1, IL-2, IL-3, IL-4, IL-6, IFN-γ) did not affect their susceptibility to the binding and the lysis mediated by LAK-cells, with the exception of IFN-γ which displayed a significant protective effect against the lysis.

The evidence herein provided that LAK-cells generated from peripheral blood and pulmonary lymphocytes can damage normal lung fibroblasts, points out that the pathogenetic mechanisms involving this self-addressed lytic activity could account for some adverse reactions related to LAK / IL-2 immunotherapy.

F-6

Subcutaneous Recombinant Interleukin-2 (IL-2) in Treatment of Metastatic Renal Cell Cancer (MRC) and Melanoma (MM).

M. Guida, A. Latorre, A. Casamassima, I. Abbate, A. Mastria, V. Lorusso, M. De Lena
Oncology Institute, Bari, Italy

Even though the initial use of intravenous IL-2 in high-dose bolus or by continuous infusion of lower doses has been limited by serious side effects, many trials have been started to maximize therapeutic efficacy and reduce toxicity. Aim of this study was to verify the efficacy of a treatment using subcutaneous rIL-2: 9 million IU / m^2 twice daily for 2 days followed by 1.8 million IU / m^2 twice daily for 5 days weekly for 6 weeks. Responding or SD patients continued maintenance therapy at 1.8 million IU / m^2 once weekly until PRO. 15 / 18 completed the treatment and are evaluable for clinical response. Two patients (1 MM, 1 MRC) refused further treatment after 2 weeks and 1 patient (MM) after 2 doses because of acute allergy. No CR was obtained. PR (13 %) was obtained in 1 MM and 1 MRC patient lasting 3 and 4 months, respectively. SD was observed in 5 MRC patients and 3 MM patients (53 %) lasting for 6 months (median). Toxicity (n=18) was moderate with local inflammation at injection site (100 %), fever and chills (83 %), malaise (56 %), hypotension (33 %), cutaneous rash (28 %), desquamative dermatitis (33 %), oliguria (22 %), nausea and vomiting (22 %), palpitations (11 %), dyspnea (5 %), acute renal failure (5 %), acute allergy (5 %). Toxicity reversed after stopping treatment. In conclusion, rIL-2 therapy was manageable and well tolerated, permitting outpatient treatment or self-administration. Moreover, it is our opinion that in spite of the low percentage of response observed, these patients might obtain a prolonged overall survival from long-term subcutaneous rIL-2 treatment.

F-7

IFN-α and IL-2 in Metastatic Melanoma: Comparison of two Phase II Trials

U. Keilholz, C. Scheibenbogen, L. Bergmann, W. Tilgen, W. Hunstein
Dept. of Medicine, and Dept. of Dermatology, University of Heidelberg, and Dept. of Medicine, University of Frankfurt

Two subsequent cohorts of patients with metastatic melanoma were treated with a combination of Interferon-α (IFN-α) and Interleukin-2 (IL-2) according to two different schedules. Schedule A consists of IFN-α, 10 Mio. IU / m^2/ day s. c. for 5 days, followed by continuous intravenous infusion of IL-2, 1 mg / m^2 / 24 hours for five days. Schedule B consists of the same dose of IFN-α, but a modified regimen of IL-2. To improve the induction of high affinity IL-2 receptors on lymphocytes, the initial IL-2 dose was increased (1 mg / m^2 / 6 hours, followed by 1 mg / m^2 / 12 hours, and 1 mg / m^2 / 24 hours). To reduce toxicity, the dose was reduced thereafter to .25 mg / sqm / 24 hours for the following three days. Both regimens were repeated after 4 weeks.

	Schedule 1 (n=27)	Schedule 2 (n=27)
Complete remission	1 (4%)	3 (11%)
Partial remission	4 (15%)	8 (30%)
Stable disease	4 (15%)	5 (18%)
Progressive disease	18 (67%)	11 (41%)
CR+PR	5 (18%)	11 (41%)
95% conf. int. (Pearson Clopper)	6–38%	22–61%
Median survival	11 months	>14 months

In four patients, residual metastatic lesions were surgically excised and no relapse has yet been observed. Severe, often dose limiting toxicity was associated with IL-2 in schedule A, particularly hypotension and fluid retention. Toxicity was significantly reduced in schedule B. Maximal serum levels of soluble CD 25, representing the induction of high affinity IL-2 receptors were 17,022±13,070 IU / ml in patients receiving schedule A, and 31,148±4,227 IU / ml in schedule B (p .01). Serum levels of TNF-α were significantly lower in schedule B than in schedule A, as were the side effects. In summary, the toxicity of IL-2 is significantly reduced by modifying the schedule of administration, the immunologic response is enhanced, and the therapeutic efficacy is increased.

F-8

Outpatient Chemo-Immunotherapy of Advanced Malignant Melanoma

J. Atzpodien, H. Kirchner, A. Schomburg, T. Menzel, M. Ackermann, M. Fenner, A. Körfer, M. Volkenandt, H. Poliwoda
Medizinische Hochschule Hannover, and Memorial Sloan-Kettering Cancer Center, New York

Both chemotherapy and Interleukin-2 and/or Interferon-α produce objective responses in a proportion of advanced malignant melanoma patients. While duration of response to chemotherapy is short i. e., usually below 4 months, immunotherapy has resulted in a small number of long-lasting remissions in patients with metastatic melanoma.

We designed a phase II trial to evaluate potential synergism between both modalities. Patients received sequential treatment consisting of carboplatin (CBDCA, 400 mg / m^2) and dacarbazine (DTIC, 750 mg / m^2) given twice (IV bolus over 30 minutes) at a 3 week interval, followed by 6 consecutive weeks of combined Interleukin-2 (rIL-2, 2.4 – 4.8 million IU / m^2 as SC bolus 2 to 3 times daily) and Interferon-α 2 (rIFN-α, 3 – 6 million IU / m^2 as SC bolus thrice weekly). Administration of CBDCA, DTIC, rIL-2 and rIFN-α was repeated unless disease progression occurred.

Among 25 evaluable patients who received sequential chemo-immunotherapy there were 3 (12%) complete responses (CRs) with durations of 10+, 16+ and 21+ months. Partial responses (PRs) were noted in 6 (24%) patients with a median response duration of 8 (range 3-11) months. Chemotherapy was administered in an ambulatory setting with mostly moderate toxicity. Thrombocytopenia was common with a median nadir on day 18 after CBDCA; 3 patients required transfusion of thrombocytes. Nausea and vomiting due to DTIC and CBDCA were well tolerated using concomitant ondansetrone (8 mg IV). Immunotherapy was self-administered at home with mild to moderate side effects; malaise, fever, chills, nausea/vomiting, diarrhea, anorexia and arthralgias were most frequent, but spontaneously reversible after ending rIL-2 / IFN-α. A mean 85% and 89% of the projected doses of rIL-2 and rIFN-α were administered. There were no treatment-related deaths.
This sequential combination of chemotherapy and rIL-2 plus rIFN-α had at least additive therapeutic activity against metastatic malignant melanoma. The schedule produced long-lasting remissions and was overall well tolerated in the outpatient setting. This trial substantiates a potential role for low to intermediate dose immunotherapy in maintaining and/or consolidating therapeutic effects of chemotherapy in metastatic melanoma.

F-9

Cytotoxic Activity of Peripheral Blood Mononuclear Cells Following Immunotherapy with IL-2 Against Autologous Melanoma Cell Lines: Role of Intercellular Adhesion Antigens and MHC-Molecules

T. Roll, C. Scheibenbogen, U. Keilholz
Dept. of Internal Medicine, University of Heidelberg

We established two melanoma cell lines from metastases of patients priot to immunotherapy. Both cell lines contain melanin and grow in adherent layers. Patients received immunotherapy with intravenous continuous infusion of IL-2 for remaining metastases. Using the standard chromium release assay, the cytotoxic activity of peripheral blood mononuclear cells (MNC) against autologous melanoma targets was assessed prior to immunotherapy and after IL-2 treatment, and for comparison also after in vitro activation of MNC with various concentrations of IL-2. To increase expression of MHC molecules and the adhesion antigens LFA 3 and ICAM 1, melanoma cells were preincubated with IFN-α or TNF-α. These two cytokines are of special interest, since IFN-α is frequently used in combination with IL-2 for immunotherapy, and TNF-α is induced by high dose IL-2 treatment in vivo. The modulation of cell surface molecules on melanoma cells was determined by FACS-analysis.
Unstimulated MNC had almost no detectable lytic activity. After immunotherapy with IL-2, MNC exhibited cytotoxic activity against autologous melanoma cells, which could be increased by preincubation of the target cells with TNF-α, which augments the expression of ICAM 1, and to a lesser extent by IFN-α, which upregulates MHC Class I molecules. Autologous LAK-cells (cultured in the presence of 1,000 IU / ml of IL-2) had high lytic activity, which was not influenced by pretreatment of target cells with cytokines. The results demonstrate that modulation of adhesion antigens and MHC molecules on melanoma cells is of great influence on susceptibility to autologous MNC, activated by IL-2 in vivo.

F-10

Adjuvant Treatment of Locally Advanced Renal Cancer with Tumorvaccines and Low-dose Interleukin-2 and Interferon-α

H. Kirchner, E. Allhoff, A. Schomburg, U. Jonas, H. Poliwoda, J. Atzpodien
Medizinische Hochschule Hannover

Locally advanced renal cell carcinoma (pT 3 b - 4 N 0 or pTx, N +) is accompanied by a high risk of relapse in spite of initial extended surgical resection.
Given the efficacy of immunomodulatory treatment in metastatic renal carcinoma, we started a clinical trial using autologous, Newcastle disease virus (NDV) modified tumorvaccines in combination with low-dose recombinant Interleukin-2 and Interferon-α 2 b for adjuvant treatment. Thirty-one patients (11 female, 20 male; median age, 58 years, range, 28 - 71 years) with locally advanced renal cell carcinoma (pT 3 - 4, pN 0 or pN +, pM 0) received subcutaneous autologous, NDV-modified and lethally irradiated tumor cells in combination with 1.8 mio. IU recombinant Interleukin-2 and 1.0 mio. IU Interferon-α 2 b once weekly over 10 weeks. Toxicity was very mild with flu-like symptoms and fevers up to 38 °C and local inflammation at the injection site. The pathological stage was defined as pT 2 - 3 a N 1 - 2 (n=21) pT 3 b - 4 N 0 (n=4) and pT 3 b - 4 N 1 - 2 (n=6). In 27 patients the follow-up was more than 6 months with a median disease-free survival of 13+ months (range, 2 - 29+ months). In addition, 6 patients with a follow-up of less than 6 months were relapse-free. Two relapses occurred at 2 and 5 months after initiation of therapy. Both had primary lymph node involvement. In summary, the surgical adjuvant use of autologous tumorvaccines in combination with low-dose cytokines may improve relapse free survival in patients with locally advanced renal cell cancer and a randomized study is needed.

F-11

Immunologic Defenses in Cervical Cancer

C. H. Evans, A. A. Flugelman, J. A. DiPaolo
Laboratory of Biology, National Cancer Institute, Bethesda, MD, USA

Human papilloma viruses (HPV), in particular type 16, are major factors in the etiology of cervical cancer. Natural killer (NK) lymphocytes, an important defense against viral diseases, are present in most HPV associated lesions and in many cases of cervical intraepithelial neoplasia. Current investigations, however, indicate that HPV type 16 positive cervical cancer cells and HPV 16 immortalized human cervical epithelial cells which possess properties similar to cells from cervical dysplasia are resistant to lysis by NK-lymphocytes. HPV positive immortalized and carcinoma cells are sensitive to lymphokine activated killer (LAK) lymphocyte lysis. Their sensitivity can be further enhanced by treatment with leukoregulin, a cytokine secreted by lymphocytes. Combination treatment with leukoregulin and a chemotherapeutic drug, e. g. cisplatin, further enhances the sensitivity of HPV 16 infected cells to LAK-lymphocyte lysis. In contrast, combined treatment with γ-Interferon can result in decreased sensitivity of HPV infected cells to destruction by LAK-lymphocytes. ^{51}Cr-labeled HPV 16 immortalized CX 16-2 cells, CX 16-2 cells malignantly transformed by v-Ha ras (PH 1-cells), and HPV 16 positive QGU cervical carcinoma cells were treated for 1 hour with 10 nM cisplatin and 2 U leukoregulin/ml or 100 U γ-Interferon (γ-IFN) / ml. Cells were incubated for 4 hours with LAK-lymphocytes and the net release of ^{51}Cr measured. Cisplatin increased CX 16-2 and QGU sensitivity to LAK-lysis by 20% and decreased PH 1 sensitivity 30%. Leukoregulin (LR) upregulated CX 16-2 sensitivity 40%, PH 1 70%, and QGU 300%. LR and cisplatin together produced a 440% synergistic increase for CX 16-2, 240% for PH 1, and 360% for QGU-cells. γ-IFN was similar to cisplatin and in combination with cisplatin reduced sensitivity to LAK up to 40%. Combined cytokine-chemotherapeutic treatment can rapidly up- or down-regulate HPV 16 positive dysplastic or neoplastic cervical epithelial cell sensitivity to LAK-lymphocyte cytotoxicity and the addition of LR can overcome the decrease in target cell sensitivtiy to LAK-lymphocyte killing produced by cisplatin.

F-12

Cloning of Peripheral Lymphocytes in Acute Phase of Acute Myeloid Leukemia Results in Predominantly CD 3 + CD 4 + T-Cell Clones with Blast Specific Autologous Cytotoxicity

B. Jahn[a], L. Bergmann[a], K. Fenchel[a], E. Weidmann[b], U. Schwuléra[c], P. S. Mitrou[a]

[a] Dept. of Hematology and Oncology, J. W. Goethe Universität, Frankfurt/Main

[b] Cancer Institute Pittsburgh, PA, USA

[c] Biotest Pharma GmbH, Frankfurt/Main

Induction of graft versus leukemia (GVL) like reaction by Interleukin-2 (IL-2) for elimination of minimal residual disease is a new therapeutic approach in treatment of acute myeloid leukemia (AML). The present study was designed to investigate mechanisms involved in specific T-cell interactions with AML blast cells in regard to cytotoxic effects. In a first step primary T-cell lines were established in an IL-2 driven coculture system and subsequently cloned by limiting dilution. Sixty-three resulting cell lines and clones were phenotypically characterized by mAbs (CD 2, CD 3, CD 4, CD 8, DR, CD 56, TCR-α / β, TCR-γ / δ). All cells stained positively for CD 2, CD 3 and DR. The vast majority of cells stained positive for CD 4 (56 / 63) and a few for CD 8 (5 / 63). In one patient 3 clones with TCR-γ / δ could be generated, two of them negative for CD 4 as well as CD 8. Expression of CD 56 was variable. Eight clones, including 4 CD 4$^+$, 2 CD 8$^+$ and 2 TCR-γ / δ^+ clones from 2 patients were chosen for functional studies in regard to cytokine release and cytotoxic activity. No significant lysis of K 562 (NK) nor Daudi cells (unspecific LAK) could be detected. However, all clones tested exerted a cytotoxic effect on autologous blast cells. The data indicate that the mechanism underlying immunotherapeutic approaches in AML treatment with IL-2 may be the in vivo activation of blast specific cytotoxic lymphocytes.

F-13

Low-Dose Interferon-γ (IFN-γ) and Interleukin-2 (IL-2) in Childhood Acute Leukemia after Autologous Bone Marrow Transplantation (ABMT): A Phase I / II Study

H. Schmid[a], E. Baumgarten[a], H. Baurmann[b], J. Brzoska[c], C. Linderkamp[a], U. Pohl[d], W. Siegert[b], G. Henze[a]

[a] Kinderklinik der Freien Universität, Berlin

[b] Universitäts-Klinikum Rudolf-Virchow, Berlin

[c] Bioferon GmbH & Co., Laupheim

[d] DRK Niedersachsen, Springe

In relapsed acute childhood leukemia ABMT offers a chance of cure even if conventional chemotherapy fails. Relapse after ABMT, however, remains a major problem. In order to prolong or maintain remission we initiated a multicenter phase I / II trial with a combination of natural IL-2 and recombinant IFN-γ. The treatment schedule consits of 7 4-week-cycles with 3 to 9 weeks resting periods. Every cycle was started with 2 doses of IFN-γ 1.5×10^6 IU / m^2 s. c. (Bioferon) followed by low-dose IL-2 10^5 IU / m^2 s. c. (DRK-Springe) 3 times per week. Since October, 1989, 20 children in complete remission after first or multiple relapses of ALL (17) and AML (3) were enrolled. Treatment was started at a median of 48 days after ABMT (range, 21 to 88). Toxicity was mild and limited to short periods of fever, fatigue, reduced appetite and weight maintenance. None of the children had to be admitted. LAK-cell related cytotoxicity of peripheral blood mononuclear cells against the RAJI cell-line and the NK-sensitive K 562 was tested. During each cycle median specific cytotoxicity increased from 25% to 37% K 562 and from 12% to 21% against RAJI, respectively. FACScan immunophenotyping of peripheral lymphocytes was performed during 10 cycles with regard to CD 3, CD 16, CD 8, and CD 56 positive cells. We observed a slight expansion of these subsets during each cycle. Compared to a historical control group of 9 patients without IFN-γ / IL-2 treatment remission duration was prolonged in patients of the study group (97 vs. 138 days, median). Disease-free survival was estimated at 27% which is comparable to ABMT without immunomodulation. In summary, this therapy with low-dose IFN-γ / IL-2 shortly after ABMT is well tolerated and can safely be given in an outpatient setting. Higher doses may be necessary to improve results significantly.

F-14

The T-cell Receptor β Chain Variable Region Repertoire in Fresh and Cultured Lymphocytes Isolated from Human Malignant Melanomas

E. Weidmann, E. M. Elder, R. B. Herberman, M. Trucco, T. L. Whiteside

Pittsburgh Cancer Institute, Pittsburgh, PA, USA

To obtain evidence for a restricted T-cell receptor (TCR) variable β (V-β) region repertoire in tumor-infiltrating lymphocytes (TIL) obtained from malignant melanomas, quantitative PCR for the expression of TCR V-β region genes was performed in 8 samples of fresh, uncultured TIL. In addition, 5 TIL preparations were studied during long-term culture in the presence of IL-2 (6,000 IU / ml) and IL-4 (1,000 IU / ml). Total cellular RNA was reverse-transcribed into cDNA, which was subsequently amplified by PCR with 22 V-β specific primers recognizing 20 V-β families and a 3' primer annealing in the constant β region. As a reference for calculating the percentage of V-β expression, a fragment of the TCR-α chain was coamplified with each V-β gene. The 3' primers for both , V-β and C-α were labeled with ^{32}(P). The amplified products were separated on 3.5% polyacrylamide gels, dried and scanned for radioactivity on an Ambis radioanalytic imaging system. The frequency of individual V-β regions was computed from the ratio of cpm V-β: cpm C-α in relation to the sum of all 22 ratios. TIL cultured in IL-2 and IL-4 were additionally studied for surface phenotype and cytotoxicity against autologous tumor. In comparison to PBL obtained from 6 healthy donors and used as control, over- or underex-pression of certain V-β regions was observed in all 8 fresh melanoma TIL studied, ranging from 0% to 48% of the total V-β expression (range in controls: 0-14%). However, different V-β genes were used by TIL obtained from various tumors, and no V-β restriction common to all TIL was identified. One to three T-cell clones, each expressing different V-β regions outgrew between days 15 and 42 of culture. However, in 4/5 TIL, this selection involved V-β7-expressing clones at some point during culture. Autotumor specific cytotoxicity did not correlate with the frequency of V-β-7 expression in TIL cultures. These data indicate that TIL isolated from individual melanomas show restricted expression of the TCR V-β genes, possibly in response to the tumor. Upon culture in the presence of cytokines, selected TIL clones outgrow, which express V-β genes different from those on fresh oligoclonal T-cells in the tumor.

F-15

Cytokine-mediated Regulated of Integrin Receptors can Influence the Adhesion of Tumor Cells to Extracellular Matrix (ECM)

E. D. Kreuser, K. Werner, M. Streit, M. Schnepf, M. P. Königsmann, W. E. Berdel, E. Thiel

Dept. of Hematology and Oncology, Klinikum Steglitz, University of Berlin

In order to elucidate the impact of cytokines on the metastatic potential of tumor cell lines, expression and regulation of integrin receptors by rIFN-α, rTNF-α, rTGF-β, and IL-4 was studied by flow cytometry using monoclonal antibodies (mAb) specific for integrin subunits. The influence of cytokines on cell cycle phases was analyzed by mAb to proliferating cell nuclear antigen (PCNA). The function of integrin receptors was assessed by measuring attachment to laminin, collagen, fibronectin, and vitronectin using a fluorometric adhesion assay. Colon cancer cell lines (HT 29, LS 180, LoVo) expressed the collagen receptors (α_1/β_1, α_2/β_1, α_3/β_1). In contrast, the fibronectin receptors (α_4/β_1, α_5/β_1) and the vitronectin receptor (α_v/β_3) were undetectable. Breast cancer cell line MCF 7 expressed high levels of collagen (α_3/β_1) and laminin (α_6/β_1) receptor. Glioblastoma cell line U 87 MG disclosed high levels of collagen (α_3/β_1) as well as fibronectin (α_5/β_1) receptor. Furthermore, U 87 MG expressed the vitronectin receptor (α_v/β_3). TNF-α significantly increased α_v/β_1 and α_6/β_1 receptors in LS 180, while TGF-β upregulated α_2/β_1 as well as α_v/β_1 receptors. rIFN-α increased integrin expression in HT 29 and MCF 7. There was no evidence that IL-4 regulated integrin receptors in these cell lines. There was no shift of cell cycle phases by rTNF-α and rIFN-α. Constitutive adhesion to ECM-proteins differed markedly between various cell lines. In HT 29, basal adhesion was 51% to collagen, 28% to laminin, 20% to fibronectin, and 5% to vitronectin. Adhesion to laminin and collagen IV was significantly increased by TNF-α in LS 180 and MCF 7. These results demonstrate: 1. β_1 and β_3 integrin receptors are heterogeneously expressed in human tumor cell lines. 2. Cytokines can selectively regulate integrin receptors, thus influencing attachment to ECM protein. 3. Receptor modulation may have a major impact on the metastatic potential of tumor cells.

F-16

Influence of Cytokines on Adhesion and Migration of Lymphocytes through Vascular Endothelial Cells

R. A. Blaheta, M. Scholz, J. Bereiter-Hahn, A. Encke, B. H. Markus

Dept. of Surgery, Transpl.-Immunol. Laboratory, J. W. Goethe University, Frankfurt/Main

Introduction: Cytokines are known to influence the penetration of lymphocytes through vascular endothelium. To get more insights into this process an in vitro assay was established using combined phase contrast and reflection contrast microscopy (RIK).

Methods: Peripheral blood lymphocytes (PBL) were added to human umbilical-vein endothelial cell (HUVE) monolayers for different time periods (0-72 hours). The cultures were treated with the cytokines α-, β-, γ-Interferon and IL-1. RIK was used to evaluate and differentiate between adherent and migrated cells. The expression of adhesion molecules ICAM-1, ELAM-1 and VCAM-1 was examined by quantitative immunostaining.

Results: Adhesion molecule expression: Enhanced expression of ELAM-1 was measured after 4-8 hours, of VCAM-1 after 8-12 hours, of ICAM-1 after 8-72 hours. Adhesion: Cytokines did not influence the maximum adhesion rate of PBL but the beginning of the adhesion process was shortened and the percentage of firmly adherent cells enhanced. Migration: Given 3 days before PBL addition to HUVE IL-1 or γ-Interferon but not α- or β-Interferon were effective in enhancing migration. Given at the same time (short or continuous stimulus) as PBL were added to HUVE all cytokines enhanced lymphocyte migration. Maximum migration was found after 2-4 hours (IL-1), 4-8 hours (α- or β-Interferon) or 8-12 hours (γ-Interferon), respectively. Therefore ICAM-1 expression did not parallel lymphocyte penetration.

Conclusion: Different cytokines influence cellular infiltration in characteristic ways. Other additional mechanisms than enhanced ICAM-1-expression seem to be responsible for the enhanced lymphocyte migration.

F-17

Interleukin-4 (IL-4) Mediated Tumor Suppression in Nude Mice Involves Interferon-γ

G. Richter, C. Platzer, K. Überla, H. Hock, T. Diamantstein, T. Blankenstein

Inst. of Immunology, Klinikum Steglitz, Berlin

The molecular events during the anti-tumor response induced by IL-4 were investigated by quantitative PCR. The growth of Chinese hamster ovary cells transfected to produce IL-4

(CH0.T1) was strongly suppressed when injected i. p. into nude mice and was accompanied by the rapid accumulation of activated macrophages. Several mRNAs were found to be upregulated during the early phase of the anti-tumor response (IL-4 receptor, IL-5, TNF and IFN-γ). The functional relevance of the elevated mRNAs was analysed by injection of CH0.T1 cells together with anti-cytokine mAbs. In contrast to anti-IL-5 and anti-TNF mAbs, an anti-IFN-γ mAb interfered with the anti-tumor response demonstrating the involvement of IFN-γ during the IL-4-induced tumor suppression. Tumor growth in anti-IFN-γ mAb treated animals was significantly delayed in comparison to anti-IL-4 mAb treated mice suggesting that IFN-γ-independent effector cells may also be involved.

F-18

Interleukin-7 Induces CD4$^+$ T-cell-dependent Tumor Rejection

H. Hock, M. Dorsch, T. Diamantstein, T. Blankenstein
Inst. für Immunologie, Klinikum Steglitz, FU Berlin, Berlin

The potential of Interleukin-7 (IL-7) to induce an anti-tumor response in vivo was analyzed. Therefore, the IL-7 gene was expressed in the plasmacytoma cell line J558L. Although the growth of IL-7-producing cells was not retarded in vitro, the IL-7-producing cells were completely rejected upon injection into mice. Tumor rejection was observed only in syngeneic but not in nude mice. The tumor-suppressive effect could be abolished by the parallel injection of an anti-IL-7 monoclonal antibody.
Immunohistochemical analysis revealed IL-7-dependent infiltration of the tumor tissue by CD4$^+$ and CD8$^+$ T-lymphocytes, and also type 3 complement receptor-positive (CR3$^+$) cells, predominantly macrophages. Depletion of T-cell subsets in tumor-bearing mice showed the absolute dependence of the anti-tumor response on CD4$^+$ cells, whereas tumor rejection was unaffected by depletion of CD8$^+$ cells. In addition to CD4$^+$ cells, CR3$^+$ cells were also needed for tumor rejection. The anti-tumor effect of IL-7 was confirmed by expression of the IL-7 gene in a second tumor cell line of different cellular origin. Together, our results demonstrate that a high local IL-7 concentration at the tumor site obtained by tumor cell-targeted gene transfer leads to tumor rejection involving a cellular mechanism that seems to be different from the ones observed in analogous experiments with other cytokines.

F-19

Membrane-bound and Soluble IL-2 Receptor, P55 and P75 Chains, on Peripheral Blood Mononuclear Cells from Patients with Solid Malignancies[1]

G. Mantovani[a], A. Maccio[a], G. Astara[a], L. Contini[a], S. Esu[a], S. Littera[a], V. Arangio[a], P. Lai[a], E. Proto[b], A. Balestrieri[a], G. S. Del Giacco[a]
[a] Dept. of Medical Oncology
[b] Dept. of Otolaryngology, University of Cagliari, Italy

The aim of the investigation was to directly study the IL-2 receptor (IL-2R), p55 and p75 chains, either membrane-bound or soluble, on PBMC of patients with solid malignancies and, indirectly, the same patients' PBMC ability to produce IL-2. 58 cancer patients, 29 men and 29 women, were studied: Their mean age was 57.3 years, range 35–79. The tumors were generally in advanced stages and in 23 cases metastatic. PBMC proliferative response to PHA, PHA plus IL-2 and IL-2 was evaluated along with the response to PHA in presence of anti-p55, anti-p75 monoclonal antibodies or both. Moreover, membrane-bound IL-2R, p55 and p75 chains, on PHA-stimulated PBMC were detected, along with soluble IL-2R in the serum and in the culture supernatants. The conclusions suggest that in solid malignancies: The membrane-bound IL-2Rs, both p55 and p75 chains, are expressed normally, there is an high serum level of sIL-2R in culture, and there is an indirect evidence of a lack of IL-2 production. Therefore, no primary impairment of IL-2R was found in solid tumors. Moreover, in our study we have found no difference in any parameter studied between patients with and patients without metastases.

[1] Work supported by CNR, A. P. 'Clinical Applications of Oncological Research', 1991 Grant.

F-20

Cytokine-Induced Tumor Immunogenicity

F. Cavallo[a], M. Giovarelli[a], A. Gulino[b], A. Vacca[b], A. Stopacciaro[d], A. Modesti[c], G. Forni[e]
[a] University of Turin
[b] University of L'Aquila
[c] University of Chieti
[d] University La Sapienza, Rome, and
[e] Immunogenetics and Histocompatibility Center, CNR, Turin, Italy

In natural conditions, proliferating tumor cells are poorly or not at all immunogenic. Nevertheless, during the early steps of tumor recognition the presence of exogenous Interleukins (ILs), as well as ILs released by IL-gene engineered tumor cells, helps the induction of an anti-tumor immune response. These ILs do not affect tumor proliferation. Rather, tumor inhibition is the result of their interference with control mechanisms of the immune system. In the present work, to get a realistic assessment of the immunogenic potential of cytokine releasing neoplastic cells, we used an expression vector to introduce the cDNA coding for murine IL-1, IL-2, IFN-γ, and IL-4 into the cells of a spontaneous, apparently non-immunogenic murine adenocarcinoma. On comparing the oncogenicity and immunogenicity of adenocarcinoma clones releasing different amounts of cytokines, it was found that disappearance of tumorigenicity and the acquisition of immunogenicity are connected events depending on the host immune system. The efficient induction of a tumor-specific immune memory rests on CD4 T-lymphocytes, the number of transfected tumor cells used, and the amount and the combination of cytokine released. The evidence that a long-lasting tumor specific immune memory takes place following a challenge with apparently non-immunogenic adenocarcinoma cells releasing cytokines supports the notion the most tumors may become immunogenic in the presence of cytokines, and holds out the prospect of strategical employment of cytokines as a component of new tumor vaccines.

Poster Discussions

P-1

A Phase II Study of Interleukin-2 (IL-2) and α-2A-Interferon (IFN) in Advanced Sarcomas

S. Toma, MC. Barzacchi, O. Sanguineti, G. Sogno, A. Venturino, R. Palumbo, G. Melioli, R. Rosso
National Institute for Cancer Research, Genoa, Italy

14 patients with advanced soft tissue sarcomas entered an outpatient phase II study in which subcutaneous IL-2 and intramuscular IFN-α were concomitantly administered. Both cytokines were given for 5 days/week for 3 consecutive weeks followed by a 2-week period during which only IFN was administered. IFN was provided at dose of 3×10^6IU, while IL-2 doses started at 2 MIU / day / m^2 (given twice a day every 12 hours and progressively the MTD of 8 MIU / day / m^2 was reached. Toxicity was mild and correlated with IL-2 dose: In fact grade III toxicity was limited to the IL-2 dose of 6 and 8 MIU / day / m^2, while no grade IV was observed. Main side effects included fever (76.6%), fatigue (39.6%), nausea and vomiting (9.9%), hypotension (29.8%), elevated liver function tests (39.3%), mild erythema and occasionally pruritus (39%), oliguria (7.8%) anemia not requiring transfusions (34.9%), granulocytopenia (9.4%). In 7 patients evaluable for response, 5 stable diseases (SD) and 2 progressions (P) were observed. In particular in 1 patient the duration of SD is up until today 30 weeks. All treated patients had severe T-cell defects at the beginning of the therapy, and virtually 11 treated subjects significantly expanded the CD16 positive, NK-cell population, during treatment. In particular, two patients who had a prolonged SD showed very high percentages (>60%) and absolute values of peripheral blood NK-cells. This regime can be administered with minimal to modeste toxicity on ambulatory and homing bases. Further accrual is needed to evaluate the efficacy of this treatment in previously treated sarcomas.

P-2

MHC-Molecules and Immunotherapy of Malignant Melanoma

C. Scheibenbogen, U. Keilholz, J. Mytilineos, M. Manasterski, W. Tilgen, W. Hunstein
Dept. of Medicine V, Dept. of Immunology, and Dept. of Dermatology, University of Heidelberg

MHC-restricted recognition of tumor cells by cytotoxic T-lymphocytes is an important mechanism in vitro. Several HLA alleles function as restriction elements for melanoma cell recognition in vitro. We investigated whether the responsiveness of malignant melanoma (MM) to immunotherapy is associated with the HLA-type of the individual patient. 56 patients with metastatic melanoma received immunotherapy either with IL-2 and lymphokin-activated killer cells or with IFN-α and IL-2 in our institution. In 32 of these melanoma patients, including 16 responders, we determined HLA haplotypes. We compared the frequency of certain common HLA class I alleles, that have been shown to function as restriction elements, namely A2, B44, and Cw7, between responders and non-responders, melanoma controls, consisting of 76 MM patients of all stages, and 126 local blood donors. All three alleles were found to be increased in responders. HLA-B44 was present in 43.8% of responders, 14.9% of melanoma controls ($p=.016$), and 12.7% of blood donors ($p=.005$), HLA-Cw7 was present in 62.5% of responders, 32.8% of melanoma controls ($p=.029$), and 47.6% of blood donors ($p=.19$), whereas the increase in A2 was not statistically significant. Our data provide evidence that the responsiveness of malignant melanoma to immunotherapy with IL-2 is associated with certain HLA types.

P-3

Regional Adoptive Immunotherapy with IL-2 and LAK-cells for Liver Metastases

U. Keilholz, C. Scheibenbogen, P. Schlag, J. Görich, GW. Kauffmann, W. Tilgen, W. Hunstein
Depts. of Internal Medicine, Surgical Oncology, Diagnostic Radiology, and Dermatology, University of Heidelberg

A novel regional approach of adoptive immunotherapy with Interleukin-2 and lymphokine activated killer cells for the treatment of liver metastases is reported. The treatment consists of continuous infusion of Interleukin-2 i. v. or into the splenic artery, and transfer of ex vivo generated lymphokine activated killer cells into the portal vein or the hepatic artery. 12 patients with malignant melanoma, 2 with renal cell carcinoma, and 1 with thyroid carcinoma have been treated. All had progressive liver metastases. In 6 patients with liver metastases of cutaneous melanoma, 2 CR (24 and 13 + months), 2 SD (10 and 6 + months), and 2 PD were observed. No responses were observed in 6 patients with liver metastases of ocular melanoma, suggesting an immunologic difference between these two melanoma subtypes. 1 PR (6 months) and 1 SD (10 months) were achieved in 2 patients with renal cell carcinoma, and 1 SD (6 + months) in the patient with thyroid carcinoma.

Trafficking studies using indium-oxine labelled cells revealed that >80% of the LAK-cells remained in the liver after regional adoptive transfer. Evidence for the crucial role of regional cell transfer is provided by the observation in a patient with an anatomic variation of hepatic blood supply in whom we achieved complete and durable tumor regression. In this case anti-tumor responses were only observed in anatomic areas of the liver which were perfused with LAK-cells.

P-4

Production of and Response to Cytokines by Peripheral Blood Cells from Cancer Patients Receiving Natural Human Lymphocyte-derived Interleukin-2

G. Pawelec[a], U. Schwuléra[b], A. Rehbein[a], E. Schlotz[a], G. Ehninger[a]
[a] Second Department of Internal Medicine, University Medical Clinic, Tübingen
[b] Biotest Pharma GmbH, Dreieich

Lymphocyte-derived, natural, glycosylated Interleukin (IL)-2 may have different effects in vivo than the non-glycosylated recombinant (r) IL-2 hitherto employed in clinical trials. To test this, 9 tumor patients were given $3-6 \times 10^6$IU / day natural IL-2 by continuous infusion for 5 days. Plasma tumor necrosis factor-α (TNF-α) levels increased considerably during therapy, Interferon-γ (IFN-γ) very slightly, whereas IL-2-stimulated secretion of either cytokine in vitro fluctuated greatly. $CD16^+$ and $CD25^+$ cells increased and $CD45R^+$ cells decreased after treatment, consistent with significant lymphocyte activation by IL-2 in vivo. Despite this, the proliferative response of treated patients' cells as well as healthy control cells to IL-2 in vitro was inhibited by IL-4 in a dose-dependent manner. In contrast, in both treated patients and controls, the proliferative response to alloantigens in mixed lymphocyte culture (MLC) was enhanced by IL-4. However, there was a striking difference between patients and controls in response to the CD3 monoclonal antibody OKT3. Normal control cells proliferated in response to OKT3 and this was markedly enhanced by IL-4, whereas patients' cells failed to respond whether or not IL-4 was present. MHC-unrestricted cytotoxicity induced by IL-2 in vitro increased after IL-2 treatment in vivo and this was also inhibited, not amplified, by IL-4. The level of $CD8^+$ cells was and remained within the normal range during treatment, although suppressive activity generated in MLC was deficient prior to therapy. Interestingly, this normalized after therapy. These results extend studies of immunological monitoring of patients receiving IL-2, based on the first trial using natural rather than rIL-2.

P-5

No Antibody Formation in Cancer Patients Treated with Natural Interleukin-2 in Combination with Recombinant Interferon-γ

J. Knüver-Hopf[a], U. Pohl[a], E. Baumgarten[b], G. Henze[b], H. Schmid[b], H. Mohr[a]

[a] German Red Cross Blood Transfusion Service of Lower Saxony, Springe

[b] Dept. of Hematology and Oncology, Pediatric Hospital, University Medical Center Rudolf Virchow, Berlin

A phase I / II clinical trial was conducted using low doses of subcutaneous natural human Interleukin-2 (nIL-2, German Red Cross Blood Transfusion Service, Springe, FRG) and subcutaneous recombinant Interferon-γ (rIFN-γ, Bioferon GmbH, Laupheim, FRG) in patients with acute leukemia or neuroblastoma after high-dose chemotherapy with autologous bone marrow transplantation.

Formation of specific IgG and IgM antibodies to Interleukin-2 and Interferon-γ was studied in a total of 16 patients.

In this preliminary report we present the results of 8 out of 16 patients who were treated for 3–12 months.

No one developed antibodies to nIL-2 during therapy. In the sera of one patient, however, we detected IgM antibodies to the nonglycosylated species of nIL-2. These antibodies were present in samples before the start of therapy and in all samples up to 4 months later.

During therapy another patient developed IgM antibodies to a 15 kD protein contamination of the rIFN-γ preparation.

The only patient to exhibit antibodies to Interferon-γ already had IgM antibodies to the Interferon-γ dimer at the onset of therapy.

The present data have to be compared with those from an earlier study in which cancer patients were treated with recombinant Interleukin-2 in combination with recombinant Interferon-Alpha. That therapy resulted in development of IgM antibodies to Interleukin-2 in 7 out of 8 patients.

P-6

Immunological Biomarkers Modifications Induced by Subcutaneous rIL-2 Treatment in Advanced Cancer Patients

I. Abbate, M. Correale, M. D. Musci, C. D. Dragone, A. Casamassima, L. Addabbo, M. Guida, A. Latorre, M. De Lena

Oncology Institute of Bari, Italy

Since the initial reports from Rosenberg et al., a number of clinical trials have confirmed that recombinant-Interleukin-2 (rIL-2)-based immunotherapy can result in durable responses in tumors refractory to conventional therapeutic approaches. We report our experience about the serum level modifications of some immunological biomarkers induced by subcutaneous (s.c) rIL-2 treatment of advanced neoplasms. Eighteen patients with advanced renal carcinoma (11) and melanomas (7) were treated with s.c rIL-2 (Proleukin-Cetus) with 9 millions IU / mq x 2 / die for two days followed by 1.8 millions IU / mq x 2 / die for five days/week for 6 cycles. We have evaluated the modifications of the serum levels of receptor for IL-2 (sIL-2 R), the expression of lymphocytic receptor for IL-2 (IL-2 R) and the benaviour of β-2 Microglobulin (β-2 M) and Neopterin (NPT) values at the end of the 2nd and 6th cycle of treatment compared to the basal values (before any treatment). In the table are reported the increases of each immunological biomarker respect the correspondent pretreatment value:

	2nd cycle	6th cycle
s-IL-2 R	7 times +	6 times +
IL-2 R	5 times +	2 times +
β-2 M	3 times +	2 times +
NPT	7 times +	5 times +

At present we are evaluating if these modifications correspond to clinical response.

P-7

Mitogen-induced Cytokine-Secretion by Lymphocytes from Patients with Small-Cell-Lung-Cancer (SCLC) and Non-Small-Cell-Lung-Cancer (NSCLC)

J. R. Fischer, M. Schindel, N. Stein, H. Lahm, H.-G. Manke, H. Galati, P. Drings

Thoraxklinik der LVA Baden, Dept. of Medical Oncology, Heidelberg and Hoffmann La Roche, Central Research Units, Basel, Switzerland

We have found that SCLC-lines secrete factors with immunosuppressive activity. Therefore, we asked whether lymphocytes and macrophages of patients with SCLC or NSCLC show an impaired capacity to produce different cytokines after in vitro stimulation via different mitogens as compared to normal control persons. For this purpose the range of cytokine concentrations in the supernatant of mitogen-stimulated immune cells of normal volunteers has to be determined. In addition to this interindividual variance, the intraindividual variance is under investigation. Furthermore, cytokine concentrations and differential blood count are related. We use whole blood for in vitro stimulation. The cells are stimulated with different mitogens and incubated for 1–4 days. Secretion of IL-1α, IL-1β, IL-2, IFN-α, IFN-γ, TNF in the supernatant of in-vitro-stimulated cells is determined by enzyme-linked-immunosorbent-assay. Preliminary results demonstrate a certain variance in cytokine concentrations between normal individuals as well as in intraindividual comparison. Furthermore, in some SCLC patients an overall suppression of cytokine secretion may be observed. We also find that at least patients with SCLC have a reduced capacity of IL-2-secretion after in vitro stimulation. Further clinical observation will reveal correlations between the cytokine-secretion-profile and treatment outcome as well as survival time. Positive correlation would lead to requirement of routine monitoring of immune profile as an additional prognostic factor in initial tumor staging.

P-8

Characterization of Functional Receptors for IL-2 on Human Solid Tumors

E. Weidmann, S. Yasumura, H. Hirabayashi, R. B. Herberman, T. L. Whiteside

Pittsburgh Cancer Institute, USA

Growth of a human squamous cell carcinoma of the head and neck (SCCHN) established in NK-cell-depleted nude mice (Cancer Res 1990;50:3113.) was found to be inhibited after local or systemic treatment with Interleukin-2 (IL-2). This observation suggested that the tumor expressed functional receptors for IL-2 (IL-2 R). To demonstrate the presence of IL-2 R on tumor cells, monoclonal antibodies to IL-2 R-α (Tac and GL439) and IL-2 R-β (TU27 and 341) were used. Two SCCHN lines (PCI-1, PCI-50), a gastric carcinoma cell line (HR) and normal human keratinocytes in 2nd-3rd passages were shown to express IL-2 R-α (in 1-30% of cells) and IL-2 R-β (in 15-90% of cells) chains by flow cytometry following dissociation of cellular monolayers by EDTA. Expression of the genes for IL-2 R-α by tumor cells was confirmed by in situ hybridization. Also, total cellular RNA was reverse transcribed, and PCR was performed with subsequent hybridization of the amplified products to full length IL-2 R-α and IL-2 R-β ^{32}(P)-labeled cDNA probes. The presence of mRNA for IL-2 R-α and -β in tumor cells was thus confirmed. When tumor cells were incubated in vitro with increasing concentrations of IL-2, dose-dependent growth inhibition (up to 40% in SCCHN and up to 50% in HR cell lines) was consistently observed. Optimal growth inhibitory IL-2 doses were 250-900 pM for PCI-1 and 22 nM for HR. This inhibitory effect of IL-2 was completely reversed by anti-IL-2 R-β, and only partially by IL-2 R-α antibodies. Cultured keratinocytes, which also expressed IL-2 R, were not inhibited in growth by IL-2. These experiments indicated that some human solid tumors express genes for IL-2 R-α and -β and that functional IL-2 receptors present on tumor cells mediate growth inhibition. Thus, IL-2 might have a direct antineoplastic effect for some tumors in addition to immunomodulatory effects. The presence of IL-2 R on human solid tumors is important to consider for optimizing IL-2 administration to patients with cancer.

P-9

Treatment Strategies in Patients with Metastatic Renal Carcinoma

J. Atzpodien, E. Allhoff, A. Körfer, A. Schomburg, T. Menzel, J. Große, I. Dallmann, M. Fenner, W. de Riese, M. Ackermann, U. Jonas, H. Poliwoda, H. Kirchner

Dept. of Hematology/Oncology and Urology, Medizinische Hochschule Hannover

We used various outpatient regimens in the therapy of metastatic renal cell carcinoma.

Subcutaneous recombinant Interleukin-2 (rIL-2) was administered alone (n=14; 14.4-18 million IU / m^2 per day, x 2 days, followed by 3.6-4.8 million IU / m^2 per day, 5 days per week, x 6 weeks) or in combination with Interferon-α 2 b (rIFN-α) (n=50; 3-6 million IU / m^2, 3 times weekly). No objective responses were seen in patients receiving sc rIL-2 as single agent, while rIL-2 / rIFN-α combination therapy produced 5 and 9 complete (CR; lung, lymph nodes, pleural metastasis) and partial remissions (PR; lung, liver, lymph nodes, bone and others), respectively (28% response rate; 44% stable disease). Median survival from start of therapy was significantly longer (19.6 months) in rIL-2 / rIFN-α treated patients than in patients receiving rIL-2 as single agent (6.4 months; $p \leq .02$). Of 28 patients who presented with progressive disease after rIFN-α and/or rIL-2, 14 each received second line therapy consisting of sc rIFN-α (6 million IU / m^2 thrice weekly) and i. v. vinblastine (6 mg / m^2 every 3 weeks), and sc rIFN-α and 5-fluorouracil (5-FU; 750 mg / m^2 as weekly i. v. bolus), respectively. One complete (lung) and 1 partial remission (lung, pancreas) occurred in vinblastine/rIFN-α treated patients (median duration of 12 months) and 1 CR (lung) and 1 PR (lung) were seen upon 5-FU/rIFN-α treatment (median duration of 15+ months).

P-10

Daily Alternating Schedules of Interferon-α and Interleukin-2 in Advanced Renal Cell Cancer - Clinical Results and Biological Effects

H.-M. Enzinger, L. Bergmann, K. Fenchel, T. Neugebauer, B. Jahn, P. S. Mitrou

Division of Hematology, Dept. of Internal Medicine, J. W. Goethe University, Frankfurt/Main

Both Interferon-α (IFN-α) and Interleukin-2 (IL-2) have some efficacy in advanced renal cell cancer (RCC) as single agents and act synergistically on activation of cytotoxic cells in vitro. In order to reduce toxicity, we treated patients with advanced RCC in a daily alternating schedule of 10 x 10^6 IU / m^2 rIFN-α s. c. (Essex-Pharma, Munich) and 18 x 10^6 IU / m^2 rIL-2 (EuroCetus, Frankfurt) as 1-hour infusion for 14 days. This cycle was repeated after a rest of 3-4 weeks up to a maximum of 4 cycles. In a following phase II study we reduced the dosages of IFN-α to 3 x 10^6 IU / m^2 and rIL-2 to 9 x 10^6 IU / m^2.

In the first study, totally 36 patients were entered, 30 were evaluable for response. 2 / 30 achieved CR and 7 / 30 PR (CR + PR = 30%) with a remission duration of 3-22+. One CR is still ongoing.

In the second study 15 patients have been entered so far, 12 are evaluable for response. Up to now the response rate in this low-dose study is only 8% (1 / 12 PR).

In both schedules no grade IV toxicities were observed, the side effects were tolerable. No major difference between the higher and lower dosages were noted. In contrast to CIVI application of IL-2 no or only a mild capillary leak syndrome was observed. High amounts of endogenous cytokine induction as IFN-γ, TNF-α and IL-6, sRIL-2 and an upregulation of endogenous IL-2 mRNA were detected. Between responders and non-responders the only significant difference was a longer persisting lymphocytosis in responders.

P-11

Interferon-α (IFN-α) Induced Transcription of Transforming Growth Factor-β_1 (TGF-β) is Impaired by Interleukin-2 (IL-2) in vivo

B. Jahn, K. Fenchel, L. Bergmann, P. S. Mitrou
Dept. of Internal Medicine, Hematology and Oncology, J. W. Goethe University, Frankfurt/Main

Interleukin-2 (IL-2) in combination with Interferon-α has been shown to have significant anti-tumoral effects in some patients with advanced renal cell cancer or malignant melanoma. As it seems possible that this therapy is modulated by secondarily induced cytokines, we investigated transcription of TGF-β in patients undergoing immunotherapy combining daily alternating application of IFN-α and IL-2 for 14 days. When gene transcription of TGF-β was analysed by Northern blotting an induction of TGF-β gene transcription in peripheral mononuclear cells (PMN) was seen 12 hours after subcutaneous IFN-α application. The following intravenous IL-2 administration diminished the amount of TGF-β specific mRNA. In contrast to first dose effect subsequent reapplication of IFN-α did not enhance TGF-β gene transcription. Only at the end of treatment course at d15 and d22 to d28 TGF-β transcription reappeared. Our results indicate a complex regulatory effect on secondarily induced cytokines as TGF-β by immunotherapeutic approaches. The down regulation of IFN-α induced TGF-β transcription may (a) represent a positive immunregulatory effect on cytotoxic cells and (b) possibly exert a modulating effect on proliferation of neoplastic tissues during combined immunotherapy.

P-12

Tumor Necrosis Factor α (TNF-α), Interleukin-1β (IL-1β) and Interleukin-6 (IL-6)-synthesis in Human Peripheral Blood Mononuclear Cells (PBMNC) Stimulated in vivo and in vitro by Proteolytic Enzymes

L. Desser, W. Macheiner, C. Oismüller, E. Kokron, A. Rehberger
Institute of Experimental and Applied Oncology, University of Vienna, Austria

Proteolytic enzymes (Bromelain and Papain) stimulate in vitro the synthesis of TNF-α, IL-1β and IL-6 in PBMNC isolated from blood of healthy donors.
TNF-α was determined in the cell supernatant by a bioassay using the cell line L929, by a radioimmunoassay and by Western blot. IL-1β and IL-6 concentration in the supernatant was measured by a RIA.
The synthesis of these cytokines depends on time of culture and on enzyme concentration.
The enzyme-induced, TNF, IL-1β and IL-6 production in PBMNC can be synergistically stimulated by IFN-α and -γ; yet, IFNs alone do not induce TNF-α production in vitro.
However, TNF-α, IL-1 and IL-6-synthesis is inducible by IFN-γ when PBMNC are obtained from donors to whom the proteolytic enzymes had been administered orally 1–3 hours before.

P-13

Effects of Ultra-Low-Dose Cytokines Plus Tumorvaccine in Advanced Malignancies during Elimination of Immune-Suppressor-Mechanisms

T. Ahlert, S. Kohler, R. Hoffmann, G. Bastert, M. Kaufmann, R. Terinde, V. Schirrmacher, M. Rexin
Universitäts-Frauenkliniken Heidelberg and Ulm
Deutsches Krebsforschungszentrum Heidelberg
Laborgemeinschaft Limbach/Schmidt-Gayk, Heidelberg

Ultra-low-dose Interleukin-2 (IL-2)/Interferon-α (IFN-α) are candidates for enhancement of antigen-specific immuneresponses and thus for combination with tumorvaccine. However, in advanced malignancies both strategies sofar failed except for limited success in melanoma and hypernephroma. Immune-suppressor-mechanisms might be present and/or induced by therapy in addition to defects in endogenous cytokine production. This hypothesis was tested in a phase I/II trial on outpatient basis: 500 mg Cyclophosphamide (d1, i. v.), 40 mg Epirubicin (d1, i. v.), 800 mg Cimetidine (d2–26), p. o.) and 75 mg Indomethacine (d2–26, p. o.) where given as anti-suppressives in addition to 1×10^6 IU IL-2 (Cetus, 2x/d, d2–26, s. c.), 3×10^6 IU IFN (Roche, 3x/week, d2–26, s. c.) and highly purified virus-/IL-2-modified, autologous, irradiated tumor cell vaccine ($1-10 \times 10^6$ cells, d2, +/-9, +/-16, i. d.). Start of next cycle: d29 or later. 19 patients (Karnowsky score 60–100) are evaluable for side effects: only mild (grade I (-II) WHO) effects where observed with respect to fiever, chills, nausea/vomiting, seldom oral mucosal affections, leukocyte depression and liver enzyme rise. Eosinophilia up to grade III occurred. 5 patients dropped out for response evaluation because of failure to complete one treatment cycle (2, ovarian/breast) or lack of biochemically/apparatively measurable disease (3 breast). 14 patients, partly receiving further cycles of therapy are evaluable suffering from ovarian (7), breast (4), vaginal-epithelial (1) and lung adenocarcinoma (1) or osteochondrosarcoma (1). They where entered in second, third or fourth line situation. There have sofar been 4 partial (3 ovarian, 1 breast) and 2 mixed responses (vaginal/lung), 3 patients remained stable (2 ovarian, 1 breast) and 5 progressed (2 ovarian, 2 breast, 1 sarcoma). Further evaluation of the strategy in a phase II/III multicenter trial seems justified and has been initiated.

P-14

Evidence for a Specific T-Cell Response in a Metastasis of Renal Cell Carcinoma Responding to Vaccination with Irradiated Autologous Tumor Cells and Transfer of in vitro Tumor-Sensitized Lymph Node Lymphocytes

E. Weidmann, T. F. Logan, J. M. Kirkwood, T. L. Whiteside
Pittsburgh Cancer Institute, USA

Vaccination of patients with autologous tumor (AuTu) cells and subsequent adoptive transfer of in vitro sensitized autologous T-cells is a more immunotherapeutic approach to cancer treatment. This approach is based on the hypothesis that the adoptively-transferred cells mediate AuTu activity and may induce long-lasting immunologic memory for the AuTu. To test this hypothesis, we studied the T-cell receptor (TCR) β chain variable (Vβ) region repertoire in peripheral blood lymphocytes (PBL) and tumor-infiltrating lymphocytes (TIL) in a patient with von Hippel Lindau disease before, during, and after immunotherapy. The patient was vaccinated with irradiated AuTu cells isolated from a renal tumor mass. 14 days later, lymph node (LN) draining the vaccination site was removed, and lymphocytes were cultured for 2 weeks in the presence of AuTu cells and 10 IU / ml of IL-2. They were adoptively transferred with systemic IL-2 given at 30,000 IU / kg every 8 hours by bolus infusion. The TCR Vβ analysis was performed as previously described by quantitative PCR (Weidmann et al: Oncol 1991;14:171.). In addition to PBL, lymphocytes obtained from a vaccine-draining LN, a non-responding renal tumor mass, and a lung metastasis responding to treatment about 3 months after therapy were studied. Changes in the frequency of the TCR Vβ - 13.1$^+$ gene expression were observed in the course of therapy as follows: Prior to treatment and during IL-2-therapy, Vβ - 13.1$^+$ T-cells represented 0.8% and 1.5%, respectively, of total PBL-T-cells. Fresh LNL isolated from a vaccine-action-draining LN contained 5.9% of Vβ - 13.1$^+$ cells. After IL-2-therapy, Vβ - 13.1$^+$ cells increased to 5.4% in PBL. In the non-responding tumor nodule, the frequency of Vβ - 13.1$^+$ cells was 12.3%. In the responding lung nodule, which was heavily infiltrated with mononuclear cells, 28% of T-cells were Vβ - 13.1$^+$, indicating that an accumulation or expansion of Vβ - 13.1$^+$ cells occurred possibly in response to a tumor-associated antigen. This expansion of Vβ - 13.1$^+$ T-cells was associated with response in the pulmonary nodule. To determine the clonality of this Vβ - 13.1$^+$ population, cloning and sequencing of the amplified Vβ - 13.1$^+$ product is currently in progress.

P-15

Real-Time Biospecific Interaction Analysis of Immobilized Interleukin-2 Receptor β Chain Peptides with Polyclonal Antibodies

K. Schmitt[a], U. Schwuléra[e], I. Amiri[b], U. Roder[c], A. Edström[c], H. Mohr[d], M. Kloft[e]

[a] Biochemical Institute, J. W. Goethe University, Frankfurt/Main
[b] Laboratoire Altergen, Strasburg, France
[c] Pharmacia Biosystems GmbH, Business Branch Biosensor, Freiburg
[d] German Red Cross Transfusion Service, Springe
[e] Biotest Pharma GmbH, Dreiech

It was the aim of this investigation to characterize the molecular interaction of polyclonal rabbit antibodies with peptides of the extracellular part of the human Interleukin-2 receptor β-chain. For this purpose the real-time biospecific interaction analysis (BIA, Pharmacia) was used. Peptide-specific rabbit antisera were raised by immunizing the animals with peptides covalently linked to a protein carrier molecule i. e. ovalbumin. For BIA experiments the same three acidic peptides i. e. SP-08 (Ala-Val-Asn-Gly-Thr-Ser-Gln-Phe-Thr-Cys; IP 5.3), SP-09 (Cys-Leu-Glu-Thr-Leu-Thr-Pro-Asp-Thr-Gln-Tyr-Glu; IP 2.8) and SP-10 (Ser-Gln-Asp-Gly-Ala-Leu-Gln-Asp-Thr-Ser-Cys; IP 2.6) were immobilized on sensor chip CM5 via thiol groups. About 250-fmole / mm^2 peptide were fixed onto the sensor chip by a newly developed method. The rabbit anti-peptide sera bound specifically the respective peptide. Compared to controls and binding to non-relevant peptide the sensorgramm shows only background levels. Furthermore antibody binding could be almost completely inhibited in competition experiments with excess of free peptide. These data clearly show that the immobilized ligand retains its specific binding properties. This method may be a useful approach to further study and characterize antibody/antigen interaction, especially in respect to the β-chain of the IL-2 receptor.

P-16

Lymphokine Activated Killer Cells Suppress Residual Acute Myeloid Leukemia Cells in Remission

H. H. Gerhartz, H. Schmetzer, F. Mayer

Med. Dept. III, Klinikum Großhadern, University of Munich

We have developed a method to identify and quantify residual leukemia progenitor cells in complete remission of acute myeloid leukemic (AML) by immunologically staining clones cultured in agar employing an enzyme-immunoassay. Leukemic colonies (CFU-L) were specifically distinguished form normal clones by their positivity for 'blast markers' like CD 10, CD 20, and CD 34. Clones of leukemic phenotype were found in all 32 cases of AML complete remission (CR) studied at a proportion of 5 - 40%. These included 14 cases of long-term remission (>24 months). CFU-L were prognostically relevant since patients relapsing within 5 months had significantly higher numbers (p=.003). Lymphokine activated killer (LAK) cells were raised from AML-patients in CR (n=9) and at relapse (n=3) by suspension culture of peripheral blood mononuclear cells with Interleukin-2 (IL-2), 1,000 units/ml). Coculture of LAK-cells with autologous bone marrow (BM) cells obtained at the same time significantly inhibited the growth of CFU-L at BM to LAK-cell ratios of 1:2.5 and 1:5 during CR (p=.01 at one-dimensional variance analysis) but not in relapsing cases (p=.28). Normal myeloid clones (CD 15-positive) were inhibited at a lesser extent only. These data show that CR of AML is a balance of normal and leukemic hematopoieses rather than eradication of leukemia which is maintained by the cytotoxic action of LAK-cells.

P-17

Immunological Changes after Interleukin-2-therapy in Patients Affected by Hematological Malignancies who Undergo Autologous Stem Cell Transplantation

A. De Laurenzi[a], V. Zoli[a], P. Iudicone[b], M. Guglielmetti[b], A. Pescarollo[a], C. Papetti[a], P. Lapponi[b], R. Scocchera[b], L. Pacilli[a], F. Blandino[a], N. Petti[a], L. Quintiliani[b]

[a] Divisione di Ematologia, Ospedale S. Camillo, Rome,
[b] Centro Nazionale Trasfusione Sangue, C. R. I., Rome, Italy

To improve the immune responsiveness of patients submitted to chemotherapy and an intensive conditioning regimen, Interleukin-2- (IL-2-) therapy was administered as three courses and the immune responses were monitored before and following every IL-2 cycle. Ten patients with hematological malignancies (5 MM, 3 NHL, 1 ALL, 1 AML), in first remission, were included in this study. IL-2 was given as a 6 day continuous infusion with escalating doses starting from 200 μg / m^2 / d up to a maximum of 1,000 μg / m^2 / d. One cycle was administered following chemotherapy, just before patients were conditioned to undergo autologous stem cell trasplantation (ASCT); two cycles were repeated after ASCT and immune reconstitution, separated by a rest period ranged between 7 - 20 days, depending on patient tolerance. The anti-tumor response was assessed measuring: a) the cytotoxic activity of peripheral blood lymphocytes (PBL) against K562 and Daudi cells in a chromium release assay; b) the Interferon (IFN-) and Tumor Necrosis Factor (TNF-) synthesis by in vitro cultured PBL. These immunological tests were performed the day before IL-2 administration (day 0) and repeated on days 9, 14, 21. Following every IL-2 cycle a consistent increase in both NK and LAK activities were generated, with a peak value on day 9: the highest responses were observed after the first IL-2 cycle following ASCT (mean values: 70% of lysis vs. K562 cells and 62% of lysis vs. Daudi cells). During the IL-2 treatment before ASCT, both lymphokine synthesis showed very low levels. After ASCT, both lymphokines were significantly higher; on day 14 of the first IL-2 cycle the IFN and TNF production was respectively: 132 IU / ml and 5,850 pg / ml, as mean values. The immunological changes induced during the 3 courses of IL-2 infusion, even if quantitatively different, support the hypothesis that IL-2-therapy contributes to eradicate minimal residual disease.

P-18

Interleukin-2 as Late Consolidation is a Promosing Approach in Second Remission of Acute Myelocytic Leukemia – Preliminary Results of a Phase II Study

L. Bergmann[a], K. Fenchel[a], G. Heil[b], K. Kolbe[c], E. Lengfelder[d], H. Martin[a], D. Bunjes[b], J. Lohmeier[e], P. S. Mitrou[a]
[a] Div. of Hematology, J. W. Goethe University, Frankfurt
[b] Div. of Hematology, University Hospital, Ulm
[c] Div. of Hematology, J. Gutenberg University, Mainz
[d] Div. of Hematology, University Hospital, Mannheim
[e] Dept. of Internal Medicine, University Hospital, Gießen

For elimination of minimal residual disease (MRD) in acute myelocytic leukemia (AML), the presence or induction of graft versus leukemia (GvL) like reactions may play a major role for the outcome of AML. Here, the induction of GvL-like reactions by IL-2 is an interesting approach for the prolongation of disease-free survival.

We conducted a multicenter phase II trial in patients with de novo AML in first relapse with an induction therapy consisting out of 2 cycles iHD-AraC (2 x 600 mg / m^2 d 1–4) and VP-16 (100 mg / m^2 d 1–7). Patients achieving CR receive a 3rd cycle as early consolidation. After a rest of 4 weeks, patients with CR receive 4 cycles rIL-2 (Euro Cetus, Frankfurt, FRG) with a dosage of 9 x 10^6 IU / m^2 d 1–5, 8–12. The cycles were repeated every 6th week. Patients undergoing autologous-BMT receive rIL-2 with the same schedule starting latest 6 weeks after a-BMT. Up to now, 9 patients could be included into the IL-2 consolidation therapy, 3 / 9 after a-BMT. The remission duration so far is 2+–27+ months, the mean is not yet reached. 3 / 9 patients exceeded their 1st relapse free intervall. Two patients relapsed after 5 and 11 months.

The toxicities were moderate, so that rIL-2 could be applicated in selected patients in an outpatient manner. However, two transplanted patients revealed sepsis and bacterial pneumonia, respectively, after IL-2-therapy.

In conclusion, this approach is practicable and the preliminary results of this still ongoing study are promising.

P-19

Upregulation of Adhesion Molecules by Immunotherapy as a Mechanism of Cytotoxocity in Renal Cell Cancer, Malignant Melanoma, and AML

K. Fenchel, L. Bergmann, B. Jahn, P. S. Mitrou
Div. of Hematology, Dept. of Internal Medicine, J. W. Goethe University, Frankfurt/Main

Adhesion molecules are a heterogenous group of surface receptors involved in cell-cell-interaction. Several cytokines including IL-1, IL-4, IL-7, TNF, and IFN-γ are able to upregulate the expression of the adhesion molecules LFA 1 and ICAM-1. The influence of IL-2 on the expression of these molecules is still uncertain.

In this study the effect of α-IFN and IL-2 on the expression of LFA 1-α, LFA 1-β, VLA 1, and ICAM-1 was investigated in 4 patients with metastatic renal cell cancer, 2 patients with malignant melanoma, receiving α-IFN 3 million IU / m^2 s. c. and IL-2 9 million IU / m^2 i. v. (bolus) in a daily alternating schedule and 3 patients with AML receiving IL-2 alone. Soluble ICAM-1 was detected by ELISA. The cellular expression of LFA 1-α, LFA 1-β, VLA 1, and ICAM-1 showed no changes during treatment, but was upregulated 7–14 days after each therapy. This corresponds to other biological effects of the IL-2 / IFN-therapy like rebound lymphocytosis, which occurred also 7–14 days following therapy. Soluble ICAM-1-serum concentrations increased in some cases with a maximum on day 8 of treatment. Following IL-2 bolus sICAM-1-serum concentrations rose to a peak after 6–8 hours followed by a rapid decline.

Immunotherapy with IL-2 / α-IFN or IL-2 alone induces upregulation of adhesion molecules, which may be an important factor of cytotoxicity. It has to be clarified, whether IL-2 or secondary cytokines are responsible for this phenomenon.

P-20

Effects of Interleukin-2 (IL-2) on Hypo-gamma-Globulinemia in Common Variable Immunodeficiency (CVID)

J. A. Rump[a], A. Jahreis[a], S. R. Stecher[a], M. Schlesier[a], R. Dräger[a], W. G. Struff[b], H. H. Peter[a]
[a] University of Freiburg, Dept. of Rheumatology and Clinical Immunology
[b] Biotest Pharma, Dreieich

17 CVID-patients and 15 healthy controls were tested for IL-2, IgM- and IgG-synthesis in vitro. Peripheral blood lymphocytes (PBL) were stimulated in vitro with anti-CD3 antibodies (OKT3), Pokeweed mitogen (PWM) and Tetanus toxoid (TT). 12 out of 18 exhibited a normal to slightly reduced IL-2 production following OKT3-stimulation but 14 patients failed to produce any IL-2 in response to PWM or TT. In addition, PBL were tested for IgM- and IgG-synthesis in vitro after stimulation with either S. aureus Cowan I (SAC) plus natural-IL-2 (n-IL-2 Biotest), PWM or TT. All CVID-patients were grouped according to a modified classification scheme proposed by Webster et al. 1990. 5 patients showed no IgM- and no IgG-synthesis after SAC plus n-IL-2-stimulation (A); 4 exhibited normal IgM- but no IgG-synthesis (B), 4 synthesized IgM and IgG in response to SAC plus n-IL-2 but not in response to PWM (C1) and 5 patients showed normal IgM- and IgG-

synthesis also after PWM-stimulation (C2). 10 out of 18 CVID-patients were enrolled in a placebo controlled, double blinded, cross over therapy study. 250,000 IU of n-IL-2 were given twice weekly for 56 weeks s. c. in addition to the regular γ-globulin infusions. During the n-IL-2-therapy phase of 28 weeks, soluble IL-2 receptors remained high, while no serum IL-2 was measurable. 2 patients needed only 40 g of γ-globulines, in contrast to 140 g before therapy. An additional 3 patients had a reduced frequency of severe infections and needed less antibiotics during n-IL-2-therapy. There was no correlation between patients' IL-2-synthesis in vitro and their response to n-IL-2-therapy in vivo.

In CVID-patients IL-2-synthesis is reduced after PWM- or TT-stimulation. IgM- and IgG-synthesis in vitro after stimulation with SAC, PWM or TT is reduced. Although n-IL-2 augments IgM- and IgG-synthesis in vitro in 13 out of 17 CVID-patients, n-IL-2-therapy failed to increase IgM- and IgG-serum levels in vivo.

P-21

Cytokines Directly Affect Contractility and Stress Protein Formation of Cardiac Myocytes

I. Löw-Friedrich, D. Weisensee, P. S. Mitrou, J. Bereiter-Hahn, W. Schoeppe
Johann Wolfgang Goethe University, Frankfurt/Main

The contractility of heart cells and the de novo synthesis of stress proteins in cardiomyocytes under cytokine exposition were studied to investigate potential toxic influences of the Interleukins (IL) and tumor necrosis factor (TNF) on the myocardium.

The contractility of cultured fetal mouse cardiac myocytes was determined in a microscope perfusion apparatus. The image of the heart cells was registered by video devices and submitted to real-time subtraction; the resulting data were operated by an image analysis system. The formation of stress proteins was monitored by an incubation of the heart cells with the test substances and subsequent labeling with L-(^{35}S) methionine. The proteins were precipitated and separated by SDS polyacrylamide gel electrophoresis. The de novo formed stress proteins were identified by autoradiography.

Under control conditions, perfused cardiac myocytes were rhythmically and synchronously contractile for many hours. IL-1 (1,000 IU / ml) caused arrhythmias resulting in a complete cessation of contractions. Perfusion with low-dose IL-2 (1,000 IU / ml) also lead to the development of arrhythmias; higher concentrations of IL-2 (100,000 IU / ml) induced complete contraction inhibition. Comparable results were registered under perfusion with IL-3 (50,000 - 100,000 IU / ml) and TNF (10,000 IU / ml). All the reported effects were reversible. Exposition to IL-1 (500 - 5,000 IU / ml) stimulated the formation of 2 stress proteins of the 70 kD molecular weight group and additionally a 30 kD protein. This stress protein was also induced by an incubation of the heart cells with IL-2 (6,000 - 50,000 IU / ml), IL-3 (300 - 10,000 IU / ml), IL-6 (2,500 - 20,000 IU / ml), and TNF (250 - 2,000 IU / ml) to a similar quantitative extent. Our results prove a direct interference of the Interleukins and TNF with cultured cardiac myocytes.

P-22

Effect of Silica on the Release of Cytokines and the Cytokine-binding Protein α-Macroglobulin from Human Monocytes

R. Frank[a], G. Birkenmeier[b], T. Walther[a], G. Kopperschläger[b], U.-F. Haustein[a]
[a] Dept. of Dermatology,
[b] Institute of Biochemistry, University of Leipzig

Long-term exposure to silica may induce silicosis and/or extra-pulmonary diseases such as scleroderma. Activated macrophages, monocytes and T-lymphocytes are involved in the early inflammatory stage of scleroderma. They are capable to release different soluble factors such as cytokines and cytokine-binding proteins that modulate fibroblast metabolism, B-cell activation and endothelial cell function. We investigated the basal secretion of cytokines (IL-1, IL-6, TNF) and cytokine-binding protein α-2-macroglobulin by human monocytes and the effect of silica on monocytes in cell culture.

In patients with scleroderma we found a slight decrease in IL-1 basal secretion from monocytes in comparison to healthy volunteers but no changes in IL-6 and TNF production. This is paralleled by a basal secretion of α-2-macroglobulin being totally transformed into the proteinase-complexed form.

Exposure by silica in monocyte-enriched cultures revealed a dose dependent modulation of the cytokine pattern. This also induces a several-fold increase in secretion of native but uncomplexed α-2-macroglobulin. The significance of α-2-macroglobulin release for cytokine function and distribution is discussed. The impact of silica on immune competent cells might explain inflammatory tissue reaction and increased collagen synthesis in silica associated scleroderma.

P-23

Treatment with Interferon-α2b, 5-Fluorouracil and Folinic Acid: Effects on Cell Surface Marker Expression in the Blood

J. Thies[a], C. Stoffregen[a], O. Stremme[a], G. Leimenstoll[b]
[a] Dept. of General Surgery,
[b] Dept. of Internal Medicine, Kiel

Interferon-α2b (IFN) is able to improve the effect of 5-Fluorouracil (5-FU) in palliative chemotherapy of gastrointestinal cancer. The immunological modulation by IFN during this treatment is still under discussion. Changes in leucocyte cell surface marker expression in blood using 7 different monoclonal antibodies were observed by fluorescence activated cell sorting. Leucocytes, CD2-, CD3-, CD4-, CD8-, CD19-, HLA-DR-antigen positive lymphocytes and natural killer cells were studied before and during chemotherapy. 15 patients with metastatic disease were treated with 3x5 Mio. IFN s. c. weekly; they received an intravenous induction therapy of 400 mg / sqm 5-FU and 200 mg / sqm FA daily during the first 6 days, then subsequent weekly maintenance treatment at the same concentrations. Leukocytes cell numbers were within the normal range prior and during chemotherapy. In general prior to treatment lymphocyte cell numbers were lowered to the half of the standard amount. This reduction was not influenced further by the chemotherapy regiment. No significant change in cell surface marker expressions of the above described antigens occurred during chemotherapy. Gastrointestinal cancer is associated with reduced lymphocyte cell numbers in our study. Combined biomodulation with IFN does not influence the measurable immunological parameters in the blood.

P-24

Intralesional Interferon-α-2b Therapy for Soft-tissue Manifestations from Malignant Melanoma

H. Voigt, R. Claßen
Melanoma Research Project, Kaltenkirchen/Holstein

Introduction: Aside from visceral metastasis, soft-tissue disease may represent the largest tumor burden in metastatic malignant melanoma thus leading to considerable patients' discomfort although not being actually course-limiting. In order to achieve tumor regression at soft-tissue sites for palliative reasons the efficacy of intralesionally (I.L.) administered Interferon-α-2b (rIFN-α2b) was piloted in a consecutive series of patients with advanced malignant melanoma presenting measurable soft-tissue lesions amenable to adjunctive I.L.-therapy.
Methods: I.L. Interferon treatment was commenced only after the patients eligible for this setting had failed to respond to systemic chemotherapy. Interferon-α-2b was administered I.L. three times weekly at a dose level of 10 Mio. IU per metastasis and a weekly maximum dose of 60 Mio. IU Dosages were subdivided into quarter parts for lesions exceeding 1.0 cm in diameter, and given as single injection for those below 1.0 cm. Administration was continued for at least 6 weeks in clockwise order according to prior mapping of metastasis. After 6 weeks of treatment patients with unresponsive lesions were excluded from further study. Evaluation of toxicity and response was performed weekly, for the latter using clinical measurements, soft-tissue ultrasound, and punch biopsy examination.
Results: So far, a total number of 44 melanoma manifestations in seven patients could be treated and assessed. I.L. Interferon therapy was well tolerated without any reasonable side effects. No toxicity WHO>2 could be encountered. Out of 44 lesions treated 24 (54.5%) regressed completely within 6 weeks of treatment. 13 lesions (29.5%) remained unchanged in size but became flattened showing no progression for 6 additional weeks. The earliest onset of regression could be assessed after 3 injections only. On biopsy, melanophagocytosis, but no residual tumor, was to be found within completely regressed lesions.
Conclusion: I.L. Interferon-α-2b appears safe and efficient for obtaining local tumor control of soft-tissue metastasis from malignant melanoma. Results achievable exceed or even match those reported from the administration of cytotoxic agents. The combination of both modalities warrant further study in order to improve on long-term palliation in this disease.

P-25

Low Relative Yield of Mononuclear Cells from Blood of Steroid-treated Glioma Patients

A. Klein-Struckmeier[a], U. Pohl[a], F. Weber[b], H. Mohr[a]
[a] German Red Cross Blood Transfusion Service of Lower Saxony, Springe
[b] Dept. of Neurosurgery, Hospital Köln/Merheim

We performed a phase I study to evaluate the safety and tolerance of local LAK/IL-2 immunotherapy for patients with high grade gliomas being currently treated with dexamthasone during immunotherapy. The relative leucocyte yield after automatic ficoll separation of leucapheresis preparations for the generation of LAK-cells was 55.8% and therefore unexpectedly low. Using the manual separation method leucocyte cell yields were only slightly different. To understand this high extent of cell loss from leucapheresis preparations which contain only small proportions of granulocytes we examined the fractionation of cells from whole blood of dexamethasone-treated glioma and non-glioma patients not involved in immunotherapy by manual method. We found that the low relative cell yield after ficoll separation is probably not glioma but corticosteroid-associated. Analysis of different bands of the gradient after separation showed that a great proportion (58% in comparison to about 30% in a healthy non-steroid treated control group) of the original mononuclear cells is enriched in the erythrocyte pellet and in the ficoll band itself. Those cells with obviously increased density are predominantly CD3/4 positive T-helper-cells which also show an intensive uptake of supravital stain.

P-26

21 KD Protein (P21) as a Marker in HIV-1-Patients During Interferon (IFN)-Therapy?

E. Grundner-Culemann[a], B. Tschechne[a], V. Neubauer[a], C. Shalitin[b], H. Poliwoda[a], I. Schedel[a], T. Benter[a]
[a] Medical School Hannover, Hannover
[b] Technion City, Haifa, Israel

Introduction: p21 is a nuclear protein frequently found in patients with proliferating urogenital, gastrointestinal tumors and HIV-1-infected patients.

Objective: To evaluate the prognostic value of p21 protein levels in patients with HIV-infection during cytokine therapy (IFN or IFN/combination).

Methods: p21 serum levels were measured monthly by ELISA in 6 HIV-infected patients during a period from 4 to 7 months (median 5.5) and compared with clinical stage (WR), disease progression and response to cytokine therapy. 3 patients suffered from Kaposi sarcoma (KS), 2 got a candida infection during therapy.

Results: In 3 patients p21 levels decreased during IFN-therapy. Constant levels were observed in 2 patients with stable disease. Changes of disease correlated with distinct increasing levels of p21 in 3 patients (1 with progress of the KS and 2 with a candida infection). After doubling the dose of IFN, start of chemotherapy and antimycotic therapy p21 level decreased again. The highest amounts of p21 were found at the beginning of IFN-therapy or in phases with opportunistic infections. The lowest amounts of p21 were observed in 1 patient without progression, which was clinical stable during long time IFN-therapy in combination with AZT.

Conclusions: Here, we detected increased levels of p21 in HIV-1-infected patients under IFN-therapy during acute infection. Protein 21 may be a useful marker for the activation of the immune system and prognostic marker during the course of IFN-therapy.

P-27

Impact of Therapy with Interferon-α-2b on Neopterin and IFN-γ Levels in Patients with Chronic Hepatitis C Virus Infection

D. Fuchs[a], G. Norkrans[b], R. Wejstal[b], G. Reibnegger[a], G. Weiss[a], O. Weiland[c], R. Schvarcz[c], A. Fryden[d], H. Wachter[a]

[a] University of Innsbruck, Austria
[b] University of Göteborg,
[c] Karolinska Institute, Göteborg,
[d] University of Linköping, Sweden

IFN-therapy was successfully applied to patients with non-A, non-B hepatitis/hepatitis C. It is still unclear whether anti-viral or immunostimulatory or both effects of IFNs are important to interfere with the disease process. In vitro, the release of neopterin from human macrophages is induced by IFNs, in particular by IFN-γ. Increased concentrations of neopterin were observed in patients with virus infections, allograft rejection, autoimmune diseases and certain types of malignancies. In addition, significant correlations between neopterin and endogenous IFN-γ existed in such patients. Likewise, therapy with IFN-α and some other cytokines like IL-2, TNF-α induce neopterin formation in patients.
In this study, serum concentrations of neopterin (by RIA, Henning) were compared to endogenous IFN-γ (by RIA, Centocor) levels in 17 patients with chronic hepatitis C before, during and after 9 months of treatment with IFN-2b.
Before therapy 10 / 17 patients had increased concentrations of neopterin and 8 had increased IFN-γ compared to healthy controls. During therapy neopterin concentrations further increased whereas IFN-γ decreased. IFN-γ and neopterin levels were correlated before ($p < .01$) but not during ($p > .1$) therapy. After end of therapy the correlation between neopterin and IFN-γ levels became again stronger.
Increased serum neopterin and IFN-γ concentrations were found in patients with chronic hepatitis C. The data indicate that increased neopterin levels is due to endogenous IFN-γ. Increase of neopterin during therapy with IFN-α appears to be due to the direct effect of IFN-α on neopterin formation.

P-28

Mechanisms of Action of Interferons on Human Malignant Glioblastoma Cell Lines

M. Doll, B. Seliger

Dept. of Hematology/Oncology, University Hospital, Mainz

Human malignant glioblastomas are the most aggressive brain tumors with poor clinical outcome. Previous studies demonstrated that autocrine growth stimulation may be the crucial event for development and maintenance of transformation of these tumors. We here show, that two malignant glioblastoma cell lines were strongly inhibited in their proliferation after IFN-α as well as IFN-γ treatment. Beside the anti-proliferative action in response to both Interferons, induction of MHC class I antigen expression and enhanced expression of Mx-A and 2'5'OASE was observed. In the presence of 20 ng / ml IFN-γ, the binding of iodinated EGF/PDGFs was strongly reduced, which was due to a specific downmodulation of receptor affinity. In contrast, treatment of the glioblastoma cell lines with 20 ng / ml IFN-α causes neither a change in growth factor receptor number nor their affinity. However, Northern and Western blot analysis revealed an induction of EGF-R mRNA after 24 hours IFN-α treatment, whereas the ligands of the EGF-R remained unaffected.
Taken together these results indicate a different mode of action of various interferons on human malignant glioblastoma cell lines. The ability of Interferons to modulate growth factor receptors has already been described as an indirect mechanism through which Interferons may affect cell growth in various systems. Further studies are in progress to investigate the signal transduction pathways of the EGF- and PDGF-systems and their possible role in growth inhibition upon Interferon treatment.

P-29

Intralesional (I.L.) Interferon Therapy for Advanced Basal Cell Carcinoma (BCC)

R. Claßen, H. Voigt, R. Bassermann

St. Bernhard-Hospital, Kamp-Lintfort

Introduction: Basal Cell Carcinoma (BCC) represents the most common skin cancer that can usually be managed curatively by resectional surgery. However, tumor dimensions, sites, and median age of the patients affected often limit invasive surgical procedures so that alternative or complementary treatment modalities warrant further study. Previous in vitro and in vivo data have demonstrated that I.L. Interferon is capable of providing local tissue concentrations high enough to induce anti-proliferative action directly at the tumor target site. Subsequently, tumor regressions can be obtained without risk of embarrassing systemic toxicity.
Methods: In a consecutive series of patients with histologically proven BCC six patients (M / F = 3 / 3; median age: 74 years) presenting 28 measurable tumor lesions were considered eligible for I.L. Interferon therapy. I.L. Interferon-α-2 a was administered at dose levels of 1.5 Mio. IU daily from D 1 through D 10 with a total dose of 15 Mio IU per lesion. Assessment of toxicity was performed daily by clinical analysis and lab count values, and response evaluation was done on day 14 and 28 using clinical analysis, photographical documentation, and histological examination.
Results: So far, 28 BCC lesions in six patients were treated. Overall toxicity was moderate and predominantly confined to inflammation at the injection site beginning on day 3 at the earliest and completely resolving after a mean duration of 10 days of continued treatment. No systemic toxicity > WHO 2 could be encountered. Clinically, out of 28 BCC lesions treated 28 disappeared completely (CR) with or immediately after completion of the protocol treatment. On biopsy, reparative fibrosis was to be found replacing BCC leaving intact epidermal structures. However, in 4 / 28 lesions reassessed histologically regrowth of BCC was seen from day 35 onwards. On the whole, tumor relapse could be found in 9 / 28 lesions treated within 16 weeks of follow-up.
Conclusion: I.L. Interferon therapy for BCC appears to be safe and efficacious for local tumor control in high risk patients not primarily amenable to invasive surgery. However, the optimal dose-response-correlation has yet to be elucidated since the observed local recurrence rate of 32% indicates inadequate loading of the tumor tissue thus providing insufficiently low local Interferon levels to induce complete regression of BCC.

Therefore, the protocol used in this series has been modified meanwhile towards injection dosages of 3 Mio. IU daily with a total loading dose of 30 Mio. IU per lesion over 10 days of treatment.

P-30

Inverse Correlation of Oncogene and MHC Class I Expression in Cells Transformed by Oncogene Inducible Expression Vectors

S. Lohmann, B. Seliger
University Hospital, Dept. of Oncology/Hematology, Mainz

Major histocompatibility complex (MHC) class I genes play a key role in immune recognition by cytotoxic T-cells. With respect to immunological surveillance an inverse relationship between MHC expression and malignancy exists. In some experimental models, MHC downregulation was strictly dependent on transformation by various oncogenes. To investigate the MHC antigen modulation in tumor cells we used a model of oncogenic transformation, in which murine fibroblasts were transfected with inducible expression vectors (MMTV-LTR) carrying the fos, mos and Ha-ras oncogene respectively. Treatment of the transfectants with dexamethasone causes colony formation in soft agar. This was associated with an increase in the fos, mos and ras oncogene expression as measured by immunofluorescence staining as well as Western blot analysis. The increase of oncogene expression was paralleled by an inhibition of MHC antigen expression. In contrast treatment of these cells with IFN-γ causes enhancement of MHC expression, whereas oncogene expression was reduced. Although MHC antigen downregulation was strictly transformation-dependent, it appeared independent of the type of oncogene causing transformation. Using the described model of oncogene inducible transformation, we would like to investigate the mechanisms of MHC downregulation.

P-31

Advantage of G-CSF in Immunoallergic Cytopenia

S. Cailleres, T. Allegre, Z. Tadrist, F. Bertucci, A. P. Blanc
Service Hématologie-Oncologie, CHG Cézanne, Aix-en-Provence, France

This report describes the cases of two female patients. The first one (44 years old) was developing a drug related tricytopenia due to Carbamizole (white cell count was 1.4×10^9 / L with 5% granulocytes and 9×10^9 / L platelets and hemoglobin was 8.6 g / dl). The other one (69 years old) a drug-related agranulocytosis (white cell count was $.8 \times 10^9$ / L with 0% granulocyte and several drugs are suspected (Allopurinol-Glibenclamide-Ticlopidine). An important infectious syndrome justified the admission.
The allergic origin was suspected because of the brutal onset and acute development of disease. Obviously, the administration of the offending drug was immediately stopped. G-CSF was rapidly introduced for a maximum of eight days. Granulocyte counts returned to the previous normal level after 9 days in the first case, and after 4 days in the second case (since G-CSF had been stopped), with respectively peak to 4,660 / mm^3 and 16,500 / mm^3. In the same way, the infectious syndrome disapeared. In the case of tricytopenia, blood platelets and hemoglobin counts returned to normal level later.
Without specific treatment, it takes about 10 days to the granulocyte count to increase of 10%. Because of G-CSF, it returned rapidly to the normal level (6.5 days); decreasing this way the infections morbidity and mortality, which is the main cause of the seriousness of this disease.

P-32

Lack of Influence of Recombinant Granulocyte Colony-stimulating Factor (G-CSF) on in vitro Growth of T-Lymphoblasts from a 5-year-old Boy with Relapse of acute Lymphoblastic Leukemia during Treatment with G-CSF

J. Greil[a], M. Peltner[a], M. Gramatzki[b], R. Burger[b], U. Kyas[c], T. Pietsch[c], J. Beck[a]
[a] Kinderklinik,
[b] Medizinische Klinik III, Universität Erlangen
[c] Kinderklinik der Medizinischen Hochschule Hannover

A 5-year-old boy with acute lymphoblastic leukemia expressing T-cell immunophenotype was treated with recombinant human G-CSF (5 μg / kg / day, s. c.) to reduce aplasia time after cytostatic treatment. During G-CSF therapy the boy relapsed with ALL. Patients leukemic blasts could be maintained in long term culture in the presence of recombinant Interleukin-7 (IL-7) for now three months. T-lymphoblasts were positive for CD 2, CD 4, CD 5 and CD 7 antigens and negative for CD 3 and CD 8. T-lymphoblasts cultured in the presence of various concentrations of G-CSF ranging from 100 ng to .1 ng per ml for four days showed no increased incorporation of ^{3}H-thymidine compared to medium controls. Moreover, specific binding sites for G-CSF on the surface of the leukemic blasts were not detectable in binding studies with ^{125}I-G-CSF. Contrasting, IL-7 induced in a concentration of 10 ng / ml a threefold increase of ^{3}H-thymidine incorporation compared to medium controls. Therefore, we conclude that in vitro recombinant human G-CSF did not induce proliferation of leukemic cells from a 5-year-old boy, who relapsed with acute lymphoblastic leukemia during treatment with G-CSF.

P-33

RH-IL-3 Opposes the Effects of Vitamins A and D on HL-60 Human Myeloid Leukemia Cells in vitro

H. R. Maurer, H. T. Hassan, C. Tsiriyotis
Institut für Pharmazie, Freie Universität Berlin

Interleukin-3 (IL-3), retinoic acid (RA) and 1.25-dihydroxyvitamin D_3 (calcitriol, vitamin D) have achieved objective responses in phase I / II clinical trials in myeloid leukemia and preleukemia patients. In order to explore any interactions between these biological agents which could provide the basis for improved therapeutic regimens for myeloid leukemia patients, we have studied the effects of IL-3 on both RA- and vitamin D-induced actions in HL-60 human myeloid leukemia cells, in both clonogenic microassays and liquid suspension cultures. The proliferative stimulus of IL-3 overrode and reversed the anti-proliferative actions of both RA and vitamin D, the latter being more sensitive to the counteracting effect of IL-3. Whereas only high concentrations of IL-3 (1,000 or more IU / m) were able to oppose the anti-proliferative effect of RA, all concentrations of IL-3 including the low concentration of 10 IU / ml significantly counteracted the anti-proliferative stimulus of IL-3 partly at low physiological and almost completely at high pharmacological concentrations. On the other hand, vitamin D prevented it only partly at high pharmacological concentrations. The same results were reproduced in liquid suspension culture. Whereas RA restrained the proliferative stimulus of IL-3, vitamin D failed to do so. However, IL-3 did not induce differentiation of HL-60 cells. The present results suggest that the clinical use of the combination of low concentrations of IL-3 with RA and not with vitamin D might restrain the progression of myeloid leukemia incurred during the treatment with IL-3 in some preleukemic patients.

P-34

Stimulation and Priming of Human Neutrophils by Granulocyte-Macrophage Colony Stimulating Factor (GM-CSF) and Poly-(Ethylene Glycol) Modified GM-CSF

M. Dómine, G. García-Manero, C. Delgado, O. P. Smith, D. Fisher, G. E. Francis

Molecular Cell Pathology Laboratory, Royal Free Hospital School of Medicine, London, UK

GM-CSF provokes direct stimulation and priming in O_2-release of human neutrophils. Attachment of poly(ethylene glycol) (PEG) to proteins improves many of their properties. We have successfully constructed biologically active PEG-GM-CSF, using a new procedure. GM-CSF and PEG-GM-CSF provoked O_2-release directly in suspended neutrophils, in a time and dose dependent manner. There was not differences between the maximal stimulation obtained with both GM-CSF and PEG-GM-CSF. However, a remarkable difference was observed in the preincubation time required for maximal stimulation, GM-CSF obtained the maximal enhancement at 30 minutes and PEG-GM-CSF at 60 minutes. To elucidate this phenomenon, we investigated the effects of GM-CSF and PEG-GM-CSF in receptor binding assays. PEG-GM-CSF binds to significantly less receptor than GM-CSF. There was, however, no significant differences in the Kd. Internalisation occurred with both cytokines but significantly more slowly with PEG-GM-CSF. PEG-GM-CSF surprisingly showed an increased activity to prime human neutrophils to respond to FMLP. The additional priming activity was time and concentration dependent. This difference was evident over a wide range of concentrations at 30 minutes, but later (80 - 120 minutes) additional activity was only seen at high concentrations. This distinctive biological activity might contribute to elucidate unexplored mechanisms for the neutrophil function.

P-35

Alternative Strategy for the Use of GM-CSF in AML: Modulation of Intracellular Ara-C Metabolism and DNA-Polymerase-α Activity in AML Blasts in vitro by GM-CSF Pretreatment

C. Reuter, U. Auf der Landwehr I, U. Auf der Landwehr II, E. Schleyer, C. Rolf, B. Wörmann, T. Büchner, W. Hiddemann

Div. of Hematology/Oncology, Dept. of Internal Medicine, University of Münster

Cytosine arabinoside (Ara-C) is one of the most active single agents in the treatment of acute myeloid leukemia (AML). Its cytotoxicity is believed to result from inhibition of DNA-synthesis and from incorporation of Ara-C into the DNA. Recent in vitro studies of our group and others indicate that pretreatment of AML blasts by hematopoietic growth factors like GM-CSF or IL-3 enhances Ara-C mediated cytotoxicity against clonogenic blasts. In order to elucidate this phenomenon we investigated the effect of GM-CSF pretreatment of AML blasts in vitro on overall DNA-polymerase, DNA-polymerase-α, thymidine and deoxycytidine kinase activity as well as ^{3}H-TdR and ^{3}H-Ara-C incorporation into the DNA. AML blasts from bone marrow (n=39 and/or peripheral blood (n=17) were incubated for 48 hours with rhGM-CSF (100 IU / ml) followed by 24 hours exposure to Ara-C at doses from .06 - 100 μM. 20 / 31 cases showed significant enhancements of ^{3}H-TdR and ^{3}H-Ara-C incorporation into the DNA (1.5 - 43.9 fold and 1.5 - 7.3 fold, respectively) in response to GM-CSF. In 10 of these 20 cases the rises in Ara-C incorporation into the DNA were only observed at low (.06 - 1 μM), and in one case only at high (1 - 100 μM) extracellular Ara-C concentrations. These enhancements correlated in 15 / 19 cases with increases in DNA-polymerase-α activity (16 - 531 %, median 72 %), in 13 / 20 cases with increases in overall DNA-polymerase activity (10 - 70 %, median 22.5 %), in 9 / 20 cases with rises of TK activity (12 - 200 %, median 27 %) and in 7 / 20 cases with enhancements of dCK activity (11 - 171 %, median 21 %) after GM-CSF. Intracellular Ara-CTP levels were not altered by GM-CSF priming. Our data suggest that GM-CSF enhances Ara-C mediated cytotoxicity in AML blasts by activition of DNA-polymerase-α and thereby increasing Ara-C incorporation into the DNA.

Acknowledgement: This work was supported by a grant from the Deutsche Krebshilfe, Dr. Mildred-Scheel-Stiftung für Krebsforschung (W 24 / 87 / Hi 1).

P-36

Discrimination of Proliferation and Antigenexpression Inducing Effects of Cytokines by Simultaneous Measurement of DNA-Content and Immunofluorescence

R. Nowak[a], U. Oelschlägel[a], T. Luther[b], I. Biester[a], H. Wolf[a]

[a] Clin. Intern. Med. Dept. Hematol./Oncol.,

[b] Inst. of Pathol., Medical Acad., Dresden

The simultaneous flow-cytometric estimation of immunophenotype and cell cycle phases is one possibility to examine various cytokine activities after short time liquid culture of bone marrow cells.

After 72 hours incubation of leukemia cells with recombinant hematopoietic growth factors in serum-free medium we have seen two effects, higher recruitment of cells in the S-phase and sometimes an increase or decrease of immunofluorescence. If the percentage of immunofluorescence positive cells after cytokine application is increased, there are two explanations: At first the cytokine has a selective proliferation inducing effect on positive cells or at the other hand the cytokine induces the expression of antigen on the cell surface. To discriminate between these two effects we propose the use of simultaneous registration of immunophenotype and DNA-content.

P-37

Pharmacodynamics of a Novel Recombinant Granulocyte Colony-stimulating Factor (rhG-CSF / BM 80.0001)

A. Sauer[a], *C. Schnell*[a], *H. Bleuel*[b], *P. Ochlich*[b], *D. B. J. Herrmann*[a], *M. Baumann*[a]
[a] Dept. of Immunopharmacology,
[b] Dept. of Pathology and Toxicology, Boehringer Mannheim GmbH

The pharmacodynamics of a novel recombinant human granulocyte colony-stimulating factor rhG-CSF / BM 80.0001 with an amino acid sequence absolutely identical to its natural counterpart has been evaluated. In in vitro models, it could be demonstrated that BM 80.0001 promotes the proliferation of a factor-dependent myeloid cell line (NFS-60) as well as the proliferation and differentiation of hematopoietic progenitor cells (CFU-C). Furthermore, BM 80.0001 enhances the functional activity of mature neutrophils (O_2-production).
In vivo, the administration of BM 80.0001 increases the leukocyte count in normal rodents and dogs in a dose-dependent manner and has marked beneficial effects on the recovery of the hematopoietic system (leukocyte count) in cyclophosphamide-pretreated animals. This pharmacological profile suggests that patients suffering from leukopenia of various origins will have a major benefit from this novel compound.

P-38

The Total Cytokine Concept: The Influence of Soluble Receptors in the Cytokine Measurement. Clinical Correlations in Pathology

D. Radoux, D. De Groote
Medgenix Diagnostics, Fleurus, Belgium

When clinical samples from different pathologies (sepsis, malaria, graft rejection, etc.) are tested with different immunoassays (commercially available or developed in house), the correlation between them is usually rather low. Furthermore, compared to the bioassays, such differences are also observed.
On the other hand, several studies showed that the membrane receptors for cytokines are released in the circulation. For example, the blood normal concentration of the two soluble TNF-α receptors is about 1 ng / ml for p 55 kD and 3 ng / ml for p 75 kD. Thus, the cytokines and their soluble receptors are present in the blood at the same time (e. g. TNF-α, IL-2, IL-1β, etc.) and both increase in some diseases.
Medgenix Diagnostics has developed the 'Total Cytokine Concept'. Non-neutralizing monoclonal antibodies have been selected and utilized to develop immunoassays. Thus, the soluble cytokine receptors have no interference in the cytokine measurement. The Medgenix cytokine immunoassays measure the total quantity of cytokines (free and bound), and not only the biologically active molecule. Correlations between the total cytokine concentration and clinical signs in different pathologies will be given.

P-39

Subcutaneous Interleukin-2 (rIL-2) and α-Interferon (rIFN-α) in Patients with Metastatic Renal Cell Cancer (RCC): A Phase II Study

R. Faggiuolo[a], *T. Borrella*[b], *D. Genesi*[c], *F. Nerva*[b], *C. Ortega*[a], *A. Prino*[d], *R. A. Antonacci*[a], *L. Dogliotti*[a]
[a] Oncologia Medica dell'Università di Torino,
[b] Divisioni di Urologia di Biella
[c] e Vercelli,
[d] Divisione di Radioterapia di Novara

In an ongoing multicenter phase II trial, 23 patients with stage IV RCC were treated with rIL-2 and rIFN-α. Their median age was 59 (36-72 years); 15 were males and 8 females; PS was 0-2 (ECOG). Patients received s. c. rIL-2 at 9-15 MU / m^2 (day 1, 2), followed by 4.5-4.8 MU / m^2 daily, 5 days a week and s. c. rIFN-α 3-6 MU / m^2 / 3 weekly, both for 6 consecutive weeks. This schedule was repeated after 2 weeks. 3 patients were early withdrawn (2 for progressive disease and 1 for toxicity). 20 patients had at least two courses of treatment and were evaluable for response. Site of metastatic disease were: Lung (9), liver (1), mixed (10). Objective response were observed in 5 patients (25%): 3 CR (15%) (13+, 12+, 6 months); 2 PR (10%) (13, 10 months). 5 patients had a stable disease and 10 (50%) progressed.
The toxicity was limited to WHO grade I and II. Local reactions at injection sites were seen in the majority of patients. Fever, anorexia and malaise occurred in all patients; none of the patients had a significant weight gain or hypotension requiring a specific therapy.
In conclusion, this therapy represents a useful regimen for patients with stage IV RCC, even if the response rate is lower than previously reported.

P-40

Subcutaneous IL-2 and Low-dose IFN-α-2A in Advanced Renal Cell Cancer: Clinical Responses and Induction of Cytokines

I. Funke, E. Späth, Schwalbe, G. Stohlmann, O. Prümmer, H. Schrezenmeier, R. Steinacker, R. Arnold, F. Porzsolt
Tumor Center and Dept. of Internal Medicine III, University of Ulm

Subcutaneous rIL-2 and low-dose rIFN-α-2 A were combined in a phase II study to evaluate efficacy, tolerance and immunological effects in unselected patients with advanced renal cell cancer. Patients were stratified to prognostic subgroups differing in ECOG status and risk factors. A high tumor burden was no reason for exclusion. One treatment cycle consisted of 18 MU IL-2 and 3 MU IFN-α on day 1-3 of week 1-3 with the fourth week off therapy. Because of toxicity WHO III and IV IL-2 doses were reduced (day 1: 18 MU, day 2: 12 MU, day 3: 6 MU) whereas IFN-α doses and the treatment rhythm were maintained. This reduced dosage regimen was tolerated in an outpatient setting. 63 treatment cycles were given to 16 patients. No remission occurred. After 3 treatment cycles, stable disease was observed in 44% of all patients and in 60% of patients with favorable prognosis.
Cytokine kinetics were determined by sandwich immuno assays during the first week of treatment. Serum levels of IL-2 and IFN-α corresponded to known pharmacokinetics. IL-6 was induced by the treatment regimen. We observed no significant induction of IFN-α and TNF-α serum levels.

P-41

Local Application of LAK-cells And nIL-2 in Malignant Glioma Therapy

F. Weber, A. Klein-Struckmeier, T. Volgmann, H. Mohr, U. Pohl, J. Menzel
Neurochirurgische Klinik Köln-Merheim

The effects of adjuvant therapy of malignant gliomas are still very unsatisfactory. Progress in immunology especially in enforcing cellular immunity by using different cytokines like IL-2 and Interferons offer new therapeutic modalities. Besides monoclonal antibodies lymphokine activated killer lymphocytes are one of the new approaches of adoptive immunotherapy where T-lymphocytes of the peripheral blood are incubated with nIL-2. Because of the results of Jacobs (1986), Ingram (1987), Merchant (1988, 1990) we started a pilot trial to investigate the safety and therapeutic efficacy of natural IL-2 and LAK-cells. This trial was performed with 16 patients which were devided in 3 groups. Five patients received a single local application of nIL-2 in increasing dosages from 10^4 to 10^6 units. Another group of 6 patients received LAK-cells. The third group of patients were treated by a combination of LAK-cells and the maximun tolerated dose of nIL-2.

The results show that a dose of 1,000,000 units of nIL-2 aswell as the application of 10^9 LAK-cells were well tolerated. No complications had been occurred. The investigation started in may 1990, so up to now the patients which were treated in this way showed a longer survival than the historical control group which was treated additional by radiation and chemotherapy. As a preliminary impression younger patients seem to have a better response respecting time to tumor progression. Perioperative an immunomonitoring was performed, wherby the relations within the L-cell subpopulation were estimated. Simultaneously, the expression of the IL-2 and transferin-receptor as an indicator of activity were measured. The activity of INF-α, IL-1, IL-4 in the peripheral blood was recorded preoperatively up to the 10. postoperative day.

P-42

β-Interferon and High-dose Tamoxifen in Patients with Advanced Breast Cancer

G. Sica[a], F. Buzzi[b], G. Rossi[c], F. Trippa[b], R. Trivisonne[d], L. Giustini[e], C. Scoponi[f], D. Pinaglia[g], M. Brugia[b]
[a] Dept. of Histology, Univ. Cattolica, Rome, and Oncology Service of
[b] Terni,
[c] Iesi,
[d] Ascoli Piceno,
[e] Fermo,
[f] Macerata,
[g] Foligno, Italy

Introduction: Few data are available in the literature concerning the effectiveness of β-Interferon (nIFN-β) and Tamoxifen (T) association in advanced breast cancer. A previous clinical experience was carried out in our Institutions with this combination in 43 patients with advanced breast cancer, pretreated with T (progressive: group A; partially responsive or stable: group B). The schedule employed was nIFN-β (Frone-Serono) 3×10^6 IU im. for 14 days, and subsequently, at the same dose, once a week. T (Nolvadex, ICI-Pharma) was started at 30 mg / day at 15th day. The results showed the ability of nIFN-β to overcome the clinical resistance (group A: objective response rate 24%) or to improve the responsiveness to T (group B: response rate 30%). With the aim of defining the optimal dose of T and timing of nIFN-β, we started, in February 1991, a phase II study with β-IFN and high-dose T including 38 patients, all pretreated with T.

Materials and Methods: Patient characteristics were: Median age 64 years (47-86), 1 premenopausal and 37 postmenopausal, median PS (ECOG) 0 (0-2), ER+ 8 patients and ER unknown 30 patients. Dominant sites of disease were: Soft-tissue 9, bone 15, and viscera 14. Twenty-one patients had been pretreated with chemotherapy (1-3 regimens). Thirty had progressed with T (group A) and 8 were responsive or stable after at least 16 weeks of T (group B). Patients received nIFN-β im. 3×10^6 IU/day three times a week, and T at 60 mg/day.

Results: All patients are evaluable for toxicity and response with a median follow-up of 4 months (r.2 - 8 m). We obtained 1 complete and 7 partial remissions (response rate 22%) and 13 stable diseases. Responses were observed in both groups (14% in group A and 50% in group B) with a median duration of response of 5 months (r.3 - 8 m +). The regimen was well tolerated. Two patients showed a grade 2 gastrointestinal toxicity and one developed a local reaction after nIFN-β injection. Our results seem to confirm the efficacy of nIFN-β to overcome the clinical resistance and to improve the responsiveness to T. However, higher dose of T employed in this study does not seem to ameliorate the response rate obtained in our previous experience with standard dose.

P-43

Expression of Murine Rantes in Cultured Mesangial Cells and in Glomeruli from Kidneys with Experimentally Induced Glomerulonephritis

G. Wolf, S. Aberle, F. Thaiss, W. Schoeppe, R. A. K. Stahl
Dept. Medicine, Div. Nephrology, University of Frankfurt/Main

Human Rantes, the prototype of the intercrine-β family of small cytokines (Scy family) was initially isolated from a cDNA library enriched for T-cell specific sequences, and has been shown to be a selective chemoattractant for CD4+ lymphocytes and macrophages/monocytes (M/M). Although originally believed to be solely expressed in T-cells, we have recently cloned and characterized the murine counterpart of human Rantes using a cDNA library prepared from renal proximal tubular epithelium. To further investigate the expression of murine Rantes (muRantes) in cultured renal cells, a 430 bp EcoRI-XhoI fragment from the clone pMuR3 was used to probe Northern blots of total RNA isolated from cultured mouse and rat mesangial cells. Stripped blots were rehybridized with a probe for the housekeeping gene GAPDH to account for small RNA loading and transfer variations. 50-100 ng/ml recombinant Interleukin-8 (IL-8), or 10-500 ng / ml recombinant tumornecrosis factor α (TNF-α) for 24 hours significantly induced expression of muRantes RNA in quiescent mouse and rat mesangial cells (relative increase in mRNA levels compared to rested control cells>x200). The TNF-α-induced increase in muRantes RNA was prevented by pretreatment with a neutralizing anti-TNF-α antibody. This induction could be also confirmed by semi-quantitative cDNA amplification applying the polymerase chain reaction. Epidermal growth factor, transforming growth factor β, or angiotensin II, over a variety of concentrations, did not induce Rantes RNA in cultured mesangial cells. A polyclonal rabbit antibody, generated against a Rantes fusion protein, revealed the presence of protein product in the cytoplasma of cultured mesangial cells. Stimulation of mesangial cells with 100 ng/ml TNF-α for 24 hours demonstrated a marked increase in immunofluorescence staining for Rantes protein. In order to characterize renal Rantes expression in vivo, a chronic proliferative glomerulonephritis was induced in Wistar rats by repeated injection of anti-mesangial cell antibody. At different time points, kidneys were harvest and mRNA was isolated from single glomerular cell suspensions. Rantes expression significantly increased five days after nephritis induction, at a time of maximal glomerular M / M accumulation. Our results demonstrate, for the first time, that mesangial cells in vivo and vitro express Rantes, and that this expression is under the complex regulation of inflammatory cytokines. It is most likely that Rantes plays a pivotal role in the glomerular recruitment of M / M which is observed in many types of glomerulonephritis.

P-44

Correlation Between TGF-β Protein Levels in Supernatants of PBMC and mRNA Levels of PBMC in Systemic Vasculitis[1]

C. Szymkowiak, J. Kekow, W. L. Gross

Dept. of Clinical Rheumatology, Medical University of Lübeck, and Dept. of Medicine, Rheumaklinik Bad Bramstedt

Cytokines are important modulators of the immune system. Exact cytokine studies comprise both mRNA and protein determinations. When we studied the expression of an anti-inflammatory cytokine in primary systemic vasculitis (PSV), we focused on the question whether the bioactivity, that was measured in PBMC supernatants using the CCL64-assay, can be correlated with the TGF-β-mRNA in PBMC. TGF-β specific mRNA determination was found to be necessary because this cytokine is present in circulation mostly in the bioinactive form which may limit the interpretation of changes in patients during disease. For a more accurate determination of the amount of mRNA we developed a semi-quantitative PCR. Cytokine specific primers were synthesized on a Milligen oligonucleotidsynthesizer with MMT-Hexylamine linker at the 5' end of the primers. Biotin-NHS-ester was coupled to the primer to allow the use of a non-radioactive chemiluminescence system for detection of PCR products. mRNA was extracted from PBMC using the guanidinium thiocyanate method. mRNA was translated into cDNA with MMLV reverse transcriptase using oligo dT$_{12-18}$ as primers. PCR was performed as multiplex PCR using the expression of mRNA for glyceraldehyde-3-phosphate dehydrogenase (GA3PDH) as an internal control for mRNA extraction and reverse transcriptase reaction. PCR products were separated on 6% native acrylamide gels, blotted onto nylon membranes and visualized with a chemiluminescence assay (Stratagene Flash system). The PCR products were quantified through laser densitometry of X-ray films. The relationship between GA3PDH and TGF-β specific mRNA in normal blood donors served as an arbitrary standard, and the cytokine expression in patients with PSV was then determined as the relative change of the standard ratio.

In active PSV, we found elevated levels of bioactive TGF-β (mean of 9.6$\pm$1.5 ng/ml in Wegener's granulomatosis, after transient acidification) which correlated well with the mRNA amount. The overall increase in mRNA was weaker than the increase in bioactivity. For further studies in PSV, TGF-β determinations either by PCR or by the CCL64 assay seem to be appropriate.

[1] Supported by a grant from the BMFT FKZ 01 VM 8906/8, and the BMFT program 'Autoimmunity'

P-45

The M20 IL-1 Inhibitor Prevents and Reduces Rheumatoid Arthritis and IL-1 Induced Inflammatory Responses in vivo

V. Barak[a], D. Peritt[a], I. Flechner[a], P. Yanai[a], T. Halperin[a], C.A. Dinarello[b], A.J. Treves[a]

[a] Deparment of Oncology, Hadassah University Hospital, Jerusalem, Israel

[b] Department of Medicine, Tufts University School of Medicine, Boston, MA, USA

We reported a specific human IL-1 Inhibitor of ~50-60 MW eluted at a pI of 4.1 found to be immunogenically distinct from the IL-1ra/IRAP. In *in vitro* experiments the factor inhibited specifically IL-1 (but not IL-2, IL-6 of TNFå) induced proliferative responses of mouse thymocytes, human T cells and fibroblasts as well as PGE_2 secretion from IL-1 induced fibroblasts. *In vivo* IL-1 induced acute inflammatory responses such as elevation of fever, leukocytosis, local lymph node enlargement and foot-pad swelling, were all reduced by concomitant injection of the factor. In addition, changes in plasma levels of fibrinogen, corticosterone, Zn, Fe and Cu induced by IL-1, were reversed by the Inhibitor. Administration of CFA into Lewis rats (AA), a model for human Rheumatoid Arthritis (RA), resulted in a severe RA. The parameters investigated were: Joint swelling, peri-articular erythema, limping of the rats and histological examination. Daily administration of IL-1 Inhibitor completely abolished the appearance of AA. The effect of the IL-1 inhibitor was shown to be dose and time dependent. These results indicate that cytokine antagonists, such as the M20 IL-1 Inhibitor, may be used to reduce inflammatory and pathological processes and, therefore, may be a useful therapeutic agent in inflammatory disorders.

Author Index

Onkologie 1992;15(suppl 1):36–37

Subject Index

Onkologie 1992;15(suppl 1):38

Onkologie 1992;15(suppl 1):39–40

Ethische und rechtliche Voraussetzungen: Zur Publikation eingereichte Manuskripte müssen bei Untersuchungen an Probanden oder Patienten die Erklärung enthalten, daß das Versuchsprotokoll von einer Ethikkommission genehmigt wurde und somit den ethischen Standards der Deklaration von Helsinki 1964 entspricht. Gleichzeitig ist die Einwilligung der Versuchsperson nach Aufklärung im Text des Manuskriptes zu fixieren. Hinweise, die auf die Identität der Versuchsperson schließen lassen, sind zu vermeiden.

Tierversuchsvorhaben bedürfen gleichfalls der Genehmigung und müssen den Forderungen des Tierschutzgesetzes in seiner Fassung von 1986 entsprechen. Auf diese Genehmigung ist im Manuskript hinzuweisen. Arbeiten, die nicht aus der Bundesrepublik Deutschland stammen, müssen einen vergleichbaren Hinweis tragen.

1. **Allgemeines, Verlagsrecht**

Bitte senden Sie Ihr Manuskript direkt an den Verlag S. Karger, z.Hd. Frau Anne Schieber, Postfach 1724, D-8034 Germering/München.

Beiträge erscheinen als Übersichtsarbeiten, Originalarbeiten, laufende klinische Studien, Kurzmitteilungen, Kasuistiken, klinisch-pathologische Konferenz, Kongreßberichte, Informationen für die Klinik und Briefe an die Herausgeber.

Originalarbeiten, Übersichtsarbeiten, laufende klinische Studien, Kurzmitteilungen und Kasuistiken sind in englischer Sprache abzufassen. Alle anderen Beiträge können wahlweise in deutscher oder englischer Sprache eingereicht werden.

Das Manuskript soll in satzreifem Zustand in dreifacher Ausfertigung eingereicht werden. Die Entscheidung über die Aufnahme erfolgt aufgrund mehrerer Gutachten. Eine Kopie des Manuskripts soll grundsätzlich beim Autor verbleiben.

Typographische Gestaltung und redaktionelle Bearbeitung sind dem Verlag vorbehalten.

Die Arbeit darf nicht gleichzeitig bei einer anderen Publikation eingereicht sein. Es ist Sache des Autors, die Nachdruckerlaubnis für Abbildungen, Tabellen usw. aus anderen Publikationen zu beschaffen. Mit der Annahme des Manuskriptes zur Publikation gehen alle Rechte auf den Verlag über. Ohne schriftliche Genehmigung des Verlages dürfen diese Publikationen oder Teile daraus nicht in andere Sprachen übersetzt oder in irgendeiner Form mit mechanischen oder elektronischen Mitteln (einschließlich Fotokopie, Tonaufnahme und Mikrokopie) reproduziert oder auf einem Datenträger oder einem Computersystem gespeichert werden.

Geschützte Markennamen müssen mit einem hochgestellten ® bezeichnet werden. Die Verantwortung für die korrekte Befolgung dieser Vorschrift liegt ausschließlich beim Autor.

2. **Manuskripte**

Diese sollen in $1^1/_2$-zeiligem Abstand geschrieben sein, links und rechts einen angemessenen breiten Rand aufweisen und (einschließlich Titelseite und Literaturverzeichnis) kontinuierlich durchnumeriert sein. Folgende Gliederung wird empfohlen:

Titelseite mit Titel und Kurztitel der Arbeit in Deutsch und Englisch; Autorenangabe; Institutsangabe in der Landessprache der Autoren.

Zusammenfassung und **Schlüsselwörter** in Deutsch und Englisch. Zusammenfassungen sind zu strukturieren in: Hintergrund, Material und Methoden, Ergebnisse, Schlußfolgerungen. In die Zusammenfassung gehören keine Literaturzitate, Tabellen, Abbildungen und Abbildungs- und Tabellenhinweise sowie allgemein gehaltene Aussagen. Zu einer Arbeit gehören 3–5 Schlüsselwörter.

Textseiten der Arbeit mit Gliederung in **Einleitung, Material und Methoden** (oder: **Patientengut** und **Methoden), Ergebnisse, Diskussionen.** Fußnoten (gegebenenfalls numeriert) am unteren Rand jeder Textseite. Abkürzungen bitte möglichst sparsam verwenden. Bei speziellen Abkürzungen jeweils beim ersten Auftreten das Wort ausschreiben und die später verwendete Abkürzung in Klammern folgen lassen: z.B. Adenosin-Monophosphat (AMP).

Ethical and legal prerequisites: Manuscripts handed in for publication dealing with examinations of probands and patients must include the declaration that the trial protocol has been approved by an ethical committee and thus meets the standards of the Declaration of Helsinki (1964). At the same time the probands' informed consent has to be included in the manuscript. Informations suitable to reveal the proband's identity are to be avoided.

Planned animal experiments demand consent as well and must meet the requirements of the laws protecting animals in the version of 1986. A reference to this approval must be included in the manuscript. Articles from outside the FRG have to include a comparable notice.

1. **General Remarks – Publishing Laws**

Please send your manuscript directly to S. KARGER Publishers attn.: Mrs. Anne Schieber, P.O. Box 1724, D-8034 Germering/Munich (FRG).

Contributions are classified as review articles, original papers, ongoing clinical studies, short communications, casuistic contributions, clinical pathological conference, congress reports, clinical information and letters to the publisher.

Original papers, review articles, ongoing clinical studies, short communications and casuistic contributions must be written in English. All other contributions may be handed in optionally in German or English.

The manuscript should be submitted in triplicate, ready for printing. Acceptance of a manuscript is based on the evaluation by several referees. The author should always keep a copy of the manuscript. The publisher reserves the right to edit the manuscript and decide on the layout.

The manuscript is received with the understanding that it is not under simultaneous consideration for publication elsewhere. It is the authors responsibility to obtain permission to reproduce illustrations, tables etc. from other publishers. Once the manuscript is accepted for publication, all the rights will be retained by the publisher. The publication, or parts of it, may not be translated into other languages, or reproduced by any mechanical or electronic means (including photocopying, recording and microcopying), or stored in a retrieval system without the publisher's written permission.

Registered trade names must be marked with the superscript registration symbol ®. It is the sole responsibility of the author to ensure that this rule is followed properly.

2. **Manuscripts**

The manuscripts should be typed in a spacing of $1^1/_2$ lines with adequately wide margins (left and right). They should be consecutively numbered (including front page and reference list). We recommend the following division:

Front page with title and short title in German and English; author's name, institute name in the native language of the authors.

Summary and **Key Words** in German (translation by the editor is possible) and English. Summaries should be structured in: Background, Material and Methods, Results, Conclusions. Summaries should not include any references, tables, figures, references to figures and tables and general statements. Each article should have 3–5 key words.

Text pages should be divided into **Introduction, Materials and Methods** (optionally **Patients and Methods), Results, Discussion.** Footnotes (with numbers) are placed at the bottom of each page of the text.

Please use abbreviations as economically as possible. Special abbreviations should be written in full when first mentioned followed by the abbreviation in parenthesis, e.g. adenosine-monophosphate (AMP). Acknowledgements should be placed directly after the text, and before the list of references.

The list of references should include only the publications cited in the text. The references should be numbered according to their

Danksagungen sollten unmittelbar dem Text folgen und dem Literaturverzeichnis vorangestellt sein.

Das Literaturverzeichnis soll nur die im Text zitierten Publikationen enthalten. Die Literatur ist entsprechend der Reihenfolge im Text zu numerieren. Es sollen nur Arbeiten, die entweder publiziert oder zur Publikation angenommen sind, zitiert werden. Der Passus «in Vorbereitung» oder «persönliche Mitteilung» ist zu vermeiden.
Literaturzitate werden mit oder ohne Angabe des Erstautors in den Text eingefügt, z. B. [1] oder Romberg [1] oder Romberg et al. [1].

Zur Abfassung von Literaturzitaten gelten folgende Beispiele:

Darstellungsschema einer Zeitschriftenreferenz:
Kauffman HF, van der Heide S, Beaumont F, Blok H, de Vries K: Class-specific antibody determination against *Aspergillus fumigatus* by means of the enzyme-linked immunosorbent assay. III. Comparative study: IgG, IgA, IgM ELISA titers, percipitating antibodies and IgE binding after fractionation of the antigen. Int Arch Allergy Appl Immunol 1986;80:300–306.

Darstellungsschema einer Buchreferenz:

Hardy WD Jr, Essex M: FeLV-induced feline acquired immune deficiency syndrome: A model for human AIDS, in Klein E (ed): Acquired Immunodeficiency Syndrome. Prog Allergy. Basel, Karger, 1986, vol 37, pp 353–376.
Die Zahl von **Abbildungen und Tabellen** soll niedrig gehalten werden und darauf abzielen, den Text zu erläutern. Abbildungen werden mit (Abb. 1), Tabellen mit (Tab. 1) in den Text eingefügt. Bereits im Text genannte Zahlen bedürfen keiner Wiederholung in einer Tabelle. Umgekehrt brauchen die in Tabellen zusammengestellten Zahlen nicht im Text wiederholt zu werden. Farbabbildungen können angenommen werden, bedürfen aber eines Reproduktions- und Druckkostenzuschusses, den der Autor zu tragen hat.
Abbildungsvorlagen sind 3fach als Papierabzüge einzureichen. Vorlagen nicht aufkleben, lochen oder mit Büroklammern anheften; auf der Rückseite den Namen des Autors, den Titel des Beitrags, die Angabe, wo «oben» ist, sowie die Bildnummer angeben.
Alle Abbildungen und Tabellen sind mit einer **Legende** zu versehen. Alle Legenden einer Arbeit werden auf einer gesonderten Seite zusammengestellt. Die Legenden sind kurz und präzise zu halten und sollen die Abbildungen bzw. Tabellen vollständig erklären. Die Interpretation der Daten erfolgt nicht in der Legende, sondern ausschließlich im Text.

Autorenadresse
Postanschrift des Autors am Schluß der Arbeit vollständig angeben.

3. **Umfang von Manuskripten**
Originalarbeiten (Gliederung s.o.) sollen 10 Textseiten nicht überschreiten.
Kurzmitteilungen folgen der Gliederung von Originalarbeiten und sollen 5 Textseiten, 5 – 10 Literaturhinweise und max. 1 Abbildung und 1 Tabelle (oder wahlweise 2 Abbildungen oder Tabellen) nicht überschreiten. Schwerpunkte von Kurzmitteilungen sollen neue Ergebnisse wissenschaftlicher Arbeiten, auch in Form sogenannter vorläufiger Mitteilungen, und auch neue Studienansätze – experimentell oder klinisch – sein. Verlag und Schriftleitung wollen erreichen, daß solche Arbeiten innerhalb kürzester Zeit publiziert werden. Selbstverständlich bleibt es dem Autor überlassen, zu einem späteren Zeitpunkt eine ausführliche Fassung einzureichen. Übersichtsarbeiten folgen nicht der Gliederung von Originalarbeiten. Titelseite, Zusammenfassung und Literaturverzeichnis (s.o.) sind jedoch erforderlich.

4. **Kosten und Sonderdrucke**
Übersteigen die Kosten der Autorkorrektur 10% der Satzkosten, müssen diese dem Autor in Rechnung gestellt werden.
Dem Autor stehen 40 Gratissonderdrucke seiner Arbeit zu.

order of appearance in the text. It is recommended to quote only articles which have been either published already or accepted for publication.
Please avoid passages like 'in preparation' or 'personal communication'. Quotes from references are inserted into the text with or without the name of the first author, e. g. [1], or Romberg [1] or Romberg et al. [1]. For references the following examples are compulsury:
Outline of a magazine reference:
Kauffman HF, van der Heide S, Beaumont F, Blok H, de Vries K: Class-specific antibody determination against *Aspergillus fumigatus* by means of the enzyme-linked immunosorbent assay . III. Comparative study: IgG, IgA, IgM ELISA titers, precipitating antibodies and IgE binding after fractionation of the antigen. Int Arch Allergy Appl Immunol 1986;80:300–306.

Outline of a book reference:
Hardy WD Jr, Essex M: FeLV-induced feline acquired immune deficiency syndrome: A model for human AIDS, in Klein E (cd): Acquired Immunodeficiency Syndrome. Prog Allergy, Basel, Karger, 1986, vol 37, pp 353–376.

The number of **figures and tables** should be limited and aim to illustrate the text. Figures are listed in the text as [fig. 1], tables as [table 1]. Figures already mentioned in the text need not be repeated in a table. Accordingly, numbers used in tables need not be repeated in the text. Figures in color may be accepted, provided the author is prepared to defray the costs involved.
Do not fasten **original figures** with glue or paper clips or punch holes in them. Please state on the back the author's name, the title of the article, the 'top' instruction and the number of the figure.
All figures and tables must include a **legend**. All legends should be listed together on a separate page. Legends should be kept short and precise and should illustrate the figures and tables exhaustively. The data should not be interpreted in the legend but exclusively in the text.

Author's address
Please give the author's full address at the bottom of the article.

3. **Volume of Manuscripts**
Original papers (framework see above) should not exceed 10 text pages.
Short communications adhere to the framework of original papers and should not exceed 5 text pages, 5–10 references and a maximum of 1 figure and 1 table (optionally either 2 figures or tables). Short communications should focus on the result of scientific studies, also in the form of so called provisional reports as well as new scientific approaches either experimental or clinical. It is the publisher's and the editorial staff's aim to manage the publishing of such articles within the shortest period of time possible. It goes without saying that the author is at liberty to hand in a complete version at a later date.
Review articles do not adhere to the framework of original papers, the title page, a summary and a list of references (see above) are, however, compulsory.

4. **Costs of Reprints**
The author will be charged for corrections to the galley proofs entailing expenses in excess of 10% of the original typesetting costs. The author is entitled to 40 free reprints of his or her article.